NICU Journal
a parent's journey

parents of _____

Important Contacts

Keep this list of phone numbers next to your phone at home and add them to your cell phone contacts. You can call the neonatal intensive care unit (NICU) anytime, day or night. If the nursery staff are busy or going through a shift change, they might have to call you back. Some NICUs contact parents in other ways. Ask the NICU staff about other options.

NICU: _____

Nurse: _____

Neonatologist: _____

Baby's doctor: _____

Lactation consultant: _____

Social worker: _____

Case manager: _____

Other: _____

_____

_____

_____

_____

Contents

Congratulations on the birth of your baby!

As parents, you are important members of your baby's health care team. You have special qualities that no doctor or nurse can match, such as a deep love and bond, which your baby knows and finds calming.

You may feel overwhelmed by the whole neonatal intensive care unit (NICU) experience. Many parents and families have experienced what you're feeling. You are not alone!

We hope this journal offers support, guidance, and comfort as you record your baby's NICU journey. This journal includes information about common issues and questions at each stage of the NICU stay, tips on coping, a glossary of common terms used in the NICU, and checklists to help track your baby's progress.

The information applies to single babies, twins, and other multiples. To make reading the journal easier, the pronoun "he" is used to describe a baby. Each and every NICU situation is unique, and some of the sections in this journal may not apply to every family. Take what you need and leave the rest.

Best wishes from all of us at the American Academy of Pediatrics!

Note: Policies and procedures at your baby's NICU may be affected by what doctors and researchers learn about COVID-19 (coronavirus disease 2019). Remember to check with your baby's NICU about the latest policies and procedures. If you have any specific questions about your baby, ask your baby's doctor. For general parenting questions, visit HealthyChildren.org.

Chapter
1
Getting to Know the NICU and Your Baby

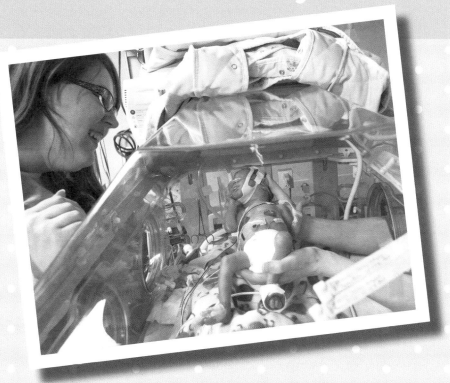

Parenting in the NICU

Every baby is a precious gift. The neonatal intensive care unit (NICU) provides the medical care for babies who are born prematurely, who are born with birth defects, or who are sick at birth. While your baby is in the NICU, your emotions can range from the joy felt over the birth of your baby and the progress being made to sadness or fear that naturally occurs when any baby is sick. It can be overwhelming!

Preterm and sick babies might not be able to handle much holding or touching at first, and they might not like loud noises or bright lights, but babies do know the voice and touch of their parents. This helps in the baby's recovery and growth.

Getting to Know the NICU Staff

The NICU doctors and nurses are here to support not only your baby but your family as well. Staff will answer questions about your baby's condition and progress and explain how the NICU works, what common NICU tests are given, and what treatments may be needed during a hospital stay. A steady exchange of information is welcomed. Feel free to ask NICU staff questions. They want to help you make the best decisions for your baby.

Your Baby's Arrival in the NICU

You can help care for your baby in the NICU from the start.

What You Can Do

- Talk with the nurses and doctors about your baby's schedule and when rounds occur.
- Ask if you can be there during medical and nursing rounds.
- Ask for a copy of the times that you can be with your baby.
- Give the NICU staff a list of phone numbers of where you can be reached. This may include home, cell, and work numbers.
- Ask about who can visit your baby in the NICU and what the visiting guidelines are.

- Let the NICU staff know how you want to receive information. This may include audio or written communication, such as printed patient handouts or videos on a Web site.

- All mothers in the NICU are encouraged to provide breast (human) milk for their babies. However, some babies may not tolerate breast milk, or it might not be safe for a mother to pump breast milk. Talk with a lactation consultant or your baby's nurse.

- Find a primary care provider, such as a pediatrician, for your baby's health care if you have not done so already. This will be your baby's main doctor after he leaves the hospital. You can ask for recommendations from the NICU staff.

- Ask what family support programs the hospital or community offers. Join a parent mentor or NICU parent support, breastfeeding support, or pumping group.

Your Baby's NICU Stay

During the NICU stay, you will learn how to care for you baby (see *Baby Care Checklist*). You may feel nervous at first, but your baby's nurses will show you what to do. Taking care of your baby may help you connect with your baby. It also will help you feel more confident of your ability to take care of your baby after leaving the NICU.

As a parent, you can give unique and loving comfort to your baby. Medical technology is important, but your little one needs your gentle touch and nurturing voice. Just as your baby is precious to you, you also are precious to your baby.

Baby Care Checklist

What You Need to Know Before Leaving the Hospital

- How to provide supportive care for your baby
- How to take your baby's temperature
- How to care for your baby's skin
- How to identify your baby's special cues
- How to care for your baby's cord area
- How to change a diaper
- How to give your baby a bath
- How to do skin-to-skin (kangaroo) care
- How to use your baby's discharge equipment, including how to tube-feed (gavage)

What You Need to Know About Your Baby

- Signs and symptoms of sickness
- Your baby's diagnoses and the plan for each diagnosis
- Medicines your baby needs and understanding side effects

If you have any questions when you get home, call the NICU, the nurse, or the discharging neonatologist.

Getting to Know Your Baby

Any baby born early (before 37 completed weeks of gestation or the 37th week of pregnancy) is considered *preterm* (you may hear such a baby referred to as *premature*, as well). The health at birth of a preterm baby (also called a *preemie*) can affect his growth and development. For example, health problems with the lungs, stomach, or brain may slow development.

The following information will show how and when the senses and sleep and wake patterns develop, and how to tell if a baby is comfortable. It also gives advice on what you can do to let your baby know you're there.

Development of Your Baby's Senses

Our senses develop before we are born. The sense of touch starts during the first trimester of pregnancy. Taste, smell, and hearing begin during the second trimester. Babies usually do not begin to see until 40 weeks' gestation. Preterm babies, depending on how early they are born, may still need to develop these senses after birth.

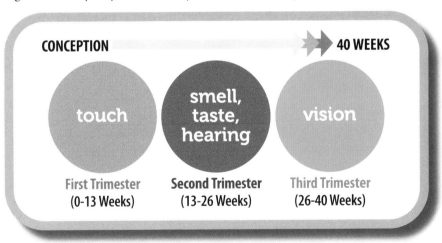

How to Let Your Baby Know You Are There

Preterm babies are very sensitive to overstimulation. Try to focus on one of your baby's senses at a time. For example, touch your baby and then talk to him—not both at the same time.

Touch

Because babies develop the sense of touch early, they are very sensitive to touch. Here are steps to help you use touch in a positive way.

- Use a constant, firm, but gentle touch. A back-and-forth touch, like stroking or massage, can be too much for a preterm baby.

- Gently cup one hand under the head and another hand on the bottoms of the feet to support a fetal position.

- Use skin-to-skin (kangaroo) care as soon as baby is ready. This can be comforting for baby and parent. Moms and dads can do skin-to-skin care with baby.

- Put your finger in your baby's hand so he can hold it.

- Your baby will get used to your touch. Always touch your baby the same way each time you greet him.

Taste and Smell

Babies use taste and smell to know who their parents are while they are in the womb. They continue to use these senses to get to know you during the NICU stay as well.

- Do not wear perfumes or scented lotions.

- Ask your doctor if it's OK to place an item that has your scent, such as a breast milk pad, scarf, or pillowcase, in your baby's incubator.

- Ask your doctor when you can start breastfeeding, if you plan on breastfeeding.

- Talk with your doctor about when to give your baby a pacifier. If you offer a pacifier, rub it a few times with your fingers so it has your scent. If you are breastfeeding, dip the pacifier in your breast milk.

- When giving your baby a pacifier, you may need to hold it in his mouth. However, take it away if he does not seem to like it.

Hearing

Babies are able to hear soft voices while they are in the womb. Talking to your baby after birth is another way for him to recognize you. The NICU is a loud place for babies, so try to avoid making unnecessary sounds.

- White-noise machines and playing music can make it harder for a baby to hear your voice.
- Keep other sounds (like closing drawers or scraping chairs) to a minimum when at your baby's bedside so your voice can be heard.
- Talk, read, or sing softly to your baby.
- Ask the nurses to help you recognize when even the sound of your voice might be too much for him.

Vision

Vision is the last sense to develop, so it needs the most protection. Very preterm babies' eyelids may still be sealed at birth but will open slowly over time. Even older babies usually need to be awake and calm for a while before they will start to use their eyes.

- Protect your baby's eyes by keeping the lights dim, covering the incubator with a blanket, and shielding his eyes from bright lights with your hands or a blanket during interaction.
- Visual stimuli, such as photos, should not be used until your baby is able to stay awake for longer periods.
- When your baby's eyes are open, keep visual stimulation simple. Your face is enough. Avoid adding more stimulation through voice or rocking when your baby's eyes are open.
- Toys placed in your baby's crib, while in the NICU, may be a potential source of infection. Also, soft objects, loose bedding, or any objects that could increase the risk of entrapment, suffocation, or strangulation should be kept out of your baby's crib. Ask your baby's health care team before adding a toy, stuffed animal, or other item to your baby's crib. See *Safe Sleep and Your Baby* in *Chapter 4, The Journey Home.*

Sleeping and Waking Time

Preterm and sick babies sleep most of the time. It is best to avoid waking them because they need sleep to grow and recover. As babies get closer to term age and get stronger, they will be able to stay awake for longer periods. Babies with health problems may not be able to increase their awake times until after their actual due date or when they get stronger.

Signs That a Baby May Be Struggling With Waking and Staying Alert

- It is hard to tell if your baby is awake or asleep. He may move around a lot and open his eyes for short periods. His eyes may move around in his head. His breathing is irregular and he often twitches and startles.

- He may wake up suddenly with a start.

- He seems fussy with no clear awake and calm periods.

- When he is awake and calm, his eyes may seem glazed or dull. He may seem panicked or worried.

- When awake and calm, he may open his eyes very wide so that they look like they are popping out. He may stare at an object and not seem to be able to look away.

- When he is awake and upset, his cry is weak and strained, and not rhythmic and robust.

- He may have trouble getting to sleep and staying asleep.

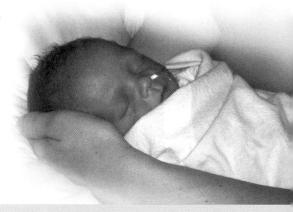

Signs That a Baby's Awake Time Is Becoming More Stable

- You can tell the difference between a light sleep and a deep sleep. During light sleep, your baby may twitch, startle, move his eyes under closed lids, and breathe irregularly, but he is clearly asleep. During deep sleep, your baby's breathing is regular, his eyes are still, and there is little movement.

- Your baby wakes up slowly with a drowsy period and his eyes open and shut over and over.

- You can tell the difference between your baby's sleeping and waking times. When he is awake, he is calm. His eyes are bright and focused and he may use eye contact to let you know he is ready to interact.

- Your baby has a strong cry.

- Your baby can calm himself by sucking on his fist or a pacifier or by hearing your voice.

Developmental Care

Preterm babies need special care and attention. Bright lights and loud noises may bother your baby, especially if he is very preterm. You also may find that your baby needs to be held or placed in certain ways. Learning the best way to care for your baby now can help him grow and develop down the road.

Lights and Sounds

Your preterm baby needs calm surroundings. You can help the NICU staff create a comfortable space for your baby by protecting your baby's eyes from bright lights. If possible, lower the lights in your baby's room. You also should avoid making loud noises around your baby and always try to speak softly to your baby.

Positioning and Holding Your Baby

It is important to provide your baby with extra support when you are positioning or holding him. Your baby's NICU team can teach you the most calming and supportive positions to place your baby. For instance, you can offer comfort and support to your baby by cradling your baby's head, bottom, or feet. These positions help your baby breathe well and help your baby's muscles develop properly. Proper positions also help your baby feel secure and lower his stress level.

Touch and Your Baby

A preterm baby's skin can be very fragile and sensitive to touch. Knowing what type of touch is best can help keep baby's skin healthy. The NICU staff will show you several ways to safely touch your baby, depending on your baby's age and size.

Constant, Steady Touch

Most preterm babies born at fewer than 26 weeks' gestation have very fragile skin and are very sensitive to touch. Don't be afraid to ask if it is OK to touch your baby. If it is not suggested at this particular time, ask when would be a good time. Once the NICU staff has told you that your baby is stable enough to touch, hold your baby's hand or let your baby hold your finger. Do not stroke, rub, or pat your baby. Instead, touch your baby gently yet steadily in the same place. Ask how often and for how long it would be best for your baby to be touched and how you will know if he needs a break.

You also can cradle your baby's head, bottom, or feet at this age. Avoid moving or rocking as you cradle your baby.

Snuggling

Even though your baby needs special kinds of touch, there are ways you can snuggle with him. Surround your baby by placing your hands close to his face and holding his knees up to his chest in a relaxed, tucked position. You can snuggle with your baby in this way while he is resting or receiving care. Snuggling can help your baby feel safe and secure.

Pain and Your Baby

If your baby shows any signs of discomfort, stop what you are doing and use your hands to cradle him in a fetal position. This is called *facilitated tucking* (or *containment*) and helps babies become calm. Babies also may use a pacifier to soothe themselves. Pay attention to how your baby reacts, as not all babies find this comforting.

Babies receive special medical care and support in the NICU. However, some procedures, such as "heel sticks" (taking blood from the baby's heel), inserting intravenous (IV) catheters (lines), injections, and removing tape from the baby's skin, can be uncomfortable. Here are some tips on how to help ease your baby's pain and discomfort during these procedures.

How can I tell if my baby is in pain or uncomfortable?

Babies cry for many reasons—they want to be changed, fed, and held—so, sometimes, it is hard to tell if a baby is in pain. The NICU staff can help you learn how to tell if your baby is uncomfortable or in pain.

Signs of pain include

- Changes in heart rate and breathing patterns
- Moving away or waving arms and legs
- Facial expressions
- Crying
- Changes in coloring and body stiffness

What can I do to make my baby more comfortable?

If your baby seems to be in pain, you can try soothing him by

- Swaddling or rocking your baby
- Placing a small drop of sucrose (a sugar solution) or a few drops of your breast milk onto your baby's tongue
- Giving your baby a pacifier, either plain or dipped in sucrose or breast milk
- Touching your baby or providing skin-to-skin (kangaroo) care
- Keeping lights and noise levels down to create a calm environment
- Talking with your doctor about pain medicines for your baby

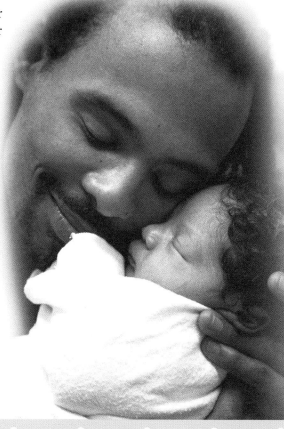

Hand Washing and Your Baby

Babies in the NICU are at risk for infections during their hospital stay. Preterm babies are at more risk because of their immature immune system and their fragile skin. Hand washing is the most important way to protect a baby. Everyone should wash their hands before and after touching your baby. Wash your hands each time you enter the nursery and anytime you have touched objects or items not located with your baby. Also wash your hands before and after you change your baby's diaper or if you touch your face or blow your nose.

The NICU will have hand-washing areas with sinks, as well as alcohol-based product dispensers throughout the unit. Alcohol-based hand sanitizers are an alternative to hand washing with soap and water. We believe they kill more germs and are less drying to hands. The NICU staff will explain what the policy is for hand washing on entry to the NICU and during your stay. Here is some important information.

On Entry to the NICU

- Remove any jewelry on your hands or wrists (you may leave a plain wedding band on).

- Place jewelry in your purse or pocket. If you cannot take your jewelry off, make sure you scrub carefully around the stones and under the bands.

- Scrub and clean for at least 20 seconds when you first enter the NICU. (As a guide, sing the ABC song twice while washing your hands.)

- Wash every part of your hands using a rubbing motion.

- Wash over and between each of your fingers, your wrist, and then up to your elbows.

- Make sure your nails and nail beds are clean.

Hand Washing in the NICU

- If you already scrubbed or washed when you entered the NICU, you can wash or use an alcohol-based product (gel) to clean your hands during your time in the NICU.

- Wash or use gel on your hands if you sneeze, cough, or blow your nose. Wash your hands before and after you change your baby's diaper.

- Wash or use gel on your hands if you touch any area of your body that has a lot of germs (your nose, mouth, face, hair, shoes) or after going to the bathroom.

- Wash or use gel on your hands between holding each baby if you have multiples.

- If you are using soap and water, place the soap on your hands and rub your hands together making a good lather.

- You must wash your hands for at least 20 seconds for germs to be killed.

- If you use the alcohol-based hand sanitizer you should get enough gel to clean your hands for 15 seconds before it dries.

Other Important Facts

- Germs love to hide under fingernails. Studies have shown that artificial nails increase the chance of infections. The NICU staff has removed theirs and it is suggested that mothers of preterm or sick babies do the same. If you do not want to remove your nails, you should consider wearing gloves before touching your baby during his hospital stay.

- It is important for you and your family to continue hand washing at home.

- Always speak out if you see anyone, even NICU staff, about to touch your baby without cleaning their hands.

Changing Your Baby's Diaper

Babies need their diapers changed several times each day. Because this requires extra touching, your baby may find it stressful. You can learn how to position and support your baby during diaper changes to help him stay calm and comfortable.

Getting Your Baby Ready for a Diaper Change

Start by gently cradling your baby's head or feet. This gentle touch can help soothe your baby. If your baby is younger than 33 weeks' gestation, place "boundaries," such as rolled blankets, around him. Support your baby's upper body by holding his arms close to his body, keeping the hands close to the face. Another way to help soothe your baby is to offer him a pacifier but only if your baby wants it.

Changing Your Baby's Diaper

Gently remove the clothes and diaper on the lower part of your baby's body. Carefully clean the skin around the diaper area and slide the new diaper under your baby. Try not to lift your baby's hips or bottom off the table or put pressure on your baby's stomach.

Some preterm babies need to rest during a diaper change to help them stay calm. The NICU staff can help you look for clues that your baby needs to take a break during a diaper change.

Always remember to wash your hands before and after a diaper change to protect you and your baby.

Skin-to-Skin (Kangaroo) Care

Skin-to-skin care (also called kangaroo care) is a special way of holding a baby against a bare chest. Holding baby close will help moms and dads feel more comfortable with their baby. The skin-to-skin contact also can improve your baby's health and development. Just ask if your baby is stable enough for you to provide skin-to-skin care. Once the NICU staff has given you the go-ahead, take full advantage of this healing touch. Be sure to take note of this special moment.

What to Do

When your baby is ready for skin-to-skin care, undress him, leaving only the diaper in place. Unbutton your shirt and place your baby on your bare chest so that his chest and stomach are touching your body. Then place a blanket over his back. Remember that you should not wear perfume or smoke cigarettes (or have the residue of secondhand smoke on your clothing or in your hair) before skin-to-skin care with your baby.

Your baby may fall asleep. The NICU staff may want to monitor your baby during this time. Skin-to-skin care can last between 1 and 2 hours. This could be a perfect opportunity to take a photograph of your baby.

What are the benefits of skin-to-skin care?

Skin-to-skin care can help your baby

- Stay warm.
- Gain weight.
- Cry less.
- Keep his heart rate, breathing, and temperature stable.
- Sleep better.
- Breastfeed better.
- Move from an incubator to a crib sooner.

Skin-to-skin care can help you

- Increase your milk production (for mothers).
- Feel more confident about caring for your baby.
- Feel a special closeness with your baby.

Feeding Your Baby

Feeding your baby is a wonderful way to feel close to your baby. Breast milk is the best first food for your baby and helps protect against infections. We encourage all mothers to pump their breast milk, whether they wish to breastfeed their baby long-term or just while their baby is in the NICU. Not every mother is able to pump her breast milk, but, if you can, it is a great way to improve your baby's health and recovery. Some hospitals offer donor breast milk. Be sure to ask your NICU staff about this.

Importance of Breast Milk

Breast milk provides many benefits for preterm and sick babies. Breast milk is tailored by your body to meet the needs of your baby. It has more proteins, and these proteins are easier for your baby to digest. It also has a higher fat content and calories for growth. Babies who are breastfed have fewer infections because of the infection-fighting immunoglobulins found in breast milk. For preterm babies, breast milk is even more important because of the still-developing intestines and kidneys. Babies who are breastfed do better, have a decreased risk of allergies, have improved eye and brain growth, and have better weight gain.

Pumping Breast Milk

Start pumping your breast milk as soon as you can after giving birth—within 6 hours if possible. This will help your body build up its milk supply. It also allows you to store your milk for your baby to use later. Your hospital will store your pumped breast milk for your baby in a safe area.

At first, try to pump every 2 to 3 hours, even at night. Try to reach a total of 100 minutes over an entire day. As your body builds up a milk supply, you may be able to reduce the number of times you need to pump each day. It is important to measure the amount of milk you produce each day. That way, you can be sure your milk supply is keeping up with your baby's needs.

Expressing Breast Milk

If you do not have access to a breast pump or need to express milk by hand, here are some tips.

- Make sure your hands are clean. Wash them well with soap and water.

- Put a clean cup or container under your breast.

- Massage the breasts gently toward the nipples.

- Place your thumb about 1 inch back from the base of the nipple and your first finger opposite.

- Press back toward your chest, and then gently compress the areola between the thumb and finger and release with a rhythmic motion until the milk flows or squirts out.

- Rotate your thumb and finger around the areola to get milk from several positions.

Transfer the milk into clean, covered containers for storage in the refrigerator or freezer. Always label and date the containers.

Early Feedings

At first, your baby may need to be fed through an IV catheter (line). But, once your baby is ready, he can be fed breast milk or formula through a small feeding tube (*gavage*). This feeding tube is inserted through the nose or mouth and goes to your baby's stomach. It can be used to feed your baby until he is ready for regular feedings by mouth.

Early feedings, often called *trophic feedings,* are provided to help your baby's intestines and prepare him for later feedings. It is important to provide breast milk for these trophic feedings if you can. The first milk your body makes is called *colostrum.* Colostrum contains many substances to protect your baby against diseases and infections. Your baby only needs a few drops, often less than a teaspoon, during the first days.

Remember, you can help with these early feedings. Talk with the NICU staff about how you can be involved. If you plan to breastfeed, ask the NICU staff how to manually express or pump your breast milk and how to store it.

Helping Your Baby Learn to Eat

Most preterm babies need help learning how to suck, swallow, and breathe at the same time. They learn to do this between 32 and 38 weeks' adjusted age (see *Chapter 7, Glossary of NICU Terms*) depending on the health and development of the baby. You can help your baby strengthen his mouth muscles by giving him a pacifier or a clean finger to suck.

As your baby grows stronger and learns to suck, you can work with the NICU staff to start feeding your baby with a bottle. Your baby still will need help with sucking, swallowing, and breathing, so take this slow. Let your baby have a few sucks at the bottle, and then let him rest and breathe for a few moments.

During these first feedings, your baby may get tired easily. Sometimes, you can help your baby eat longer by placing your finger under his chin and holding his cheeks lightly while he sucks on the bottle. Your baby's nurse can show you this technique.

Ask your baby's nurse about *cue-based feeding*. Cue-based feeding is a method of oral feeding that is based on a baby's developmental maturity. It is also called "infant-driven feeding" because feeding is based on when a baby shows readiness for oral feeding through specific behaviors or cues.

Breastfeeding

Most preterm babies cannot breastfeed right away. However, once you and your baby are ready, breastfeeding can be a wonderful experience, and you will feel good knowing that your breast milk is the best food for your baby.

When your baby is ready, hold him to your bare chest and practice skin-to-skin (kangaroo) care. Your baby will be comforted by your closeness and your milk will flow more easily. When holding your baby skin-to-skin, practice guiding him to your nipple. In time, this may help your baby "latch on" to your breast more easily.

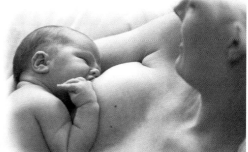

For babies not ready to breastfeed, nonnutritive breastfeeding after milk has been expressed or pumped lets them get used to the breastfeeding process.

Each breastfeeding experience is different. It may take time to adjust to your baby's feeding style. For mothers of multiples, it is important to remember that, even if your babies are identical, they will be different from each other, and each breastfeeding experience is different from baby to baby and from feeding to feeding. A lactation consultant is available at most hospitals to help new mothers with breastfeeding.

Fortifying Breast Milk

Your baby may need extra calories, proteins, and minerals for growth. Your baby's doctor may recommend that you add breast milk fortifier or formula to your breast milk.

Feeding Multiples

It is possible to breastfeed more than one baby at a time. If you decide to breast-feed your twins or triplets, here are some things you can do to make this a more positive experience.

- Work with a lactation consultant who has experience with multiples.
- Get as much sleep, food, and water as possible.
- Get tips from other mothers of multiples who have breastfed their babies.
- Have someone help position your babies when feeding 2 at a time—at least until your babies have enough neck support to move toward your breast on their own (usually when they weigh 10 lb).
- Provide skin-to-skin care with your babies as much as possible.
- Pump your breasts after breastfeeding to help increase your milk production.
- Encourage family members to learn about the benefits of breastfeeding preterm multiples so that they can offer help and support.

If you are the mother of multiples, you should ask how best you can color-code your pumped breast milk and how best to divide and store your breast milk from each pumping session, so that your baby who is healthiest and first ready to receive your breast milk will not be the only one to receive your very first and most beneficial early milk. Each of your babies, once they are ready to receive your milk, should be given your early expressed breast milk so that they will each be afforded the same benefits of this milk.

Bottle-feeding
You can connect with your baby while bottle-feeding. To make the most of your time together, hold your baby close and look into his eyes during the feeding.

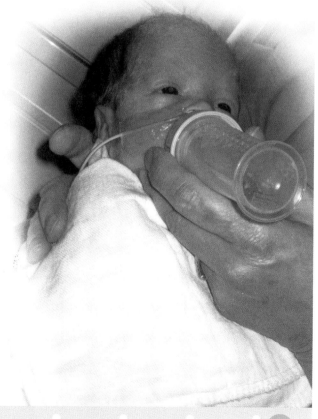

Bathing Your Baby

Preterm babies have delicate skin that requires gentle bathing styles, such as "spot" and "swaddled" bathing. Learning more about how to bathe your baby can help make it an even better experience for you both.

Spot Bathing

At first, your baby may only need to be cleaned in certain areas, such as the mouth and diaper area, and around tubes or other equipment. Simply wet a soft, smooth cloth with clean water and gently wipe the spots on your baby that need cleaning, and then dab the spots with a dry cloth.

If the NICU staff bathes your baby, ask if you can hold your baby during the bath. You also can comfort your baby during bath time by offering a pacifier or holding his finger. It is not uncommon for a baby to cry the first few times he is bathed. This is a whole new experience and new sensation for him, and it will be important to be exceptionally gentle and slow in your movements and care.

Swaddled Bathing

As your baby grows stronger, he will be ready for a swaddled bath. Wrap your baby in a blanket or cloth. Next, place your wrapped baby in a tub of warm water so that the water touches his shoulders. (Never let go during a bath.) Use a soft, smooth, wet cloth (without soap) to wash your baby's face by wiping from nose to ears. Once the face is clean, pat it dry.

After you have cleaned your baby's face, add cleansing lotion to your wet cloth. Remove one part of the blanket at a time to wash the body. Cover each area after you have washed it. Once you have washed your baby's entire body, use the soapy, wet cloth to wash the hair, and then rinse the soap from your baby's hair with clean water.

Once you have finished bathing your baby, remove him from the wet blanket and wrap him in a warm, dry towel. Cover your baby's head to keep him warm and gently pat him dry. It is not uncommon for parents to feel clumsy or all thumbs the first few times they do this. This is a totally new experience for you, and your NICU staff knows this. They are there to help and support you as you learn to care for your baby.

Most first-time mothers of term babies do not have the gift of having a professional medical staff right at their fingertips to help them maneuver through this milestone—just another gift from your preterm or sick baby! Ask someone to take a picture of you and your baby during this big event, and don't forget to note this date on your Special Moments page (see *Chapter 2, Journaling*).

Late-Preterm Babies and Multiples

A baby born 4 to 6 weeks before his due date is often referred to as a "late-preterm" baby. Even though these babies are just a few weeks early, they are prone to having their own unique early health or developmental problems. Even though a late-preterm baby may look very healthy, much like a baby born at full term, he is at much greater risk for potentially serious health problems than full-term babies. Late-preterm babies are also at higher risk for having to be readmitted to the hospital after they go home from the newborn nursery or the NICU.

What You Need to Know During the First Year

If you have a late-preterm baby, here are a few things to pay attention to during the first year. In this section, "your baby's doctor" refers to your baby's primary care provider, such as a pediatrician.

- **Feeding.** While in the hospital and after discharge, your baby may take a little longer to feed and may need to eat more often. Work with the NICU staff to develop a feeding plan before you leave the hospital. It is very important that your baby takes in enough breast milk, formula, or both, especially in the first couple days after birth when he is at greater risk for jaundice. Most mothers appreciate assistance from the lactation professional or nurse to help the baby latch on and maintain breastfeeding. Your baby may become tired and not nurse or bottle-feed very long. Ask your baby's doctor how many wet diapers a day your baby should have and how much your baby should eat.

- **Sleeping.** Initially, your baby may sleep longer than a full-term baby. It is important to make sure he eats at least every 4 hours. You may have to wake him for feedings if he is not eating frequently enough. Remember to put your baby on his back to sleep. Ask your baby's doctor how long your baby should sleep before you wake him.

- **Breathing.** A baby's lungs are one of the last parts of his body to be fully developed and, even if your baby did not need additional oxygen or a respirator, your baby's lungs are still developing. Even though your baby was born just a few weeks before his due date, his lungs are immature and very sensitive. Secondhand tobacco smoke, perfumes, and environmental pollutants can irritate your baby's airways and cause distress very easily. If your baby is having any trouble breathing, call 911 immediately, and then call your baby's doctor. In advance, remember to ask your baby's doctor what the best way is to reach him or her.

- **Clothing.** Babies born early have less body fat than full-term babies. This extra fat in the last few weeks of pregnancy is very important, and babies born even just a little early have more difficulty maintaining a normal body temperature and will lose heat very quickly. Cold, preterm babies will use their calories to stay warm and will not grow and develop like they should. It is important to keep your baby away from drafts and keep the room warmer than you might otherwise. If you are going out in colder weather or into air-conditioning, consider using a hat and blanket to help keep your baby warm. Dress your baby in one layer more than you are wearing. Ask your baby's doctor how you can best assess the appropriate layer of clothing for your baby.

- **Jaundice.** Your baby will be screened for jaundice before he goes home from the hospital, but he is still at risk for hyperbilirubinemia. Your baby will be tested for this just before discharge, and you should find out the results of the hospital screening before you go home. Visit your baby's doctor within 24 to 48 hours after your baby comes home from the hospital. If your baby's skin appears yellow or orange in color and if he is not eating well, you should call his doctor immediately. Ask your baby's doctor or nurse how to best assess your baby for jaundice.

- **Protection from infections.** Like all babies just leaving the hospital, your baby has not had all of his immunizations, and you should be careful to avoid exposing him to people with infections. Avoid going out in crowds. Late-preterm babies have an immature immune system and are at a greater risk of infection than full-term babies. Watch for signs and symptoms of infection and call your baby's doctor with any concerns. One of the best ways to avoid exposing your baby to harmful germs and viruses is through proper hand washing. Ask all visitors to wash their hands before touching your baby. Also ask visitors to postpone their visit if they are sick or have been around anyone else who is sick. Most people don't understand how fragile and vulnerable to infection your baby is, even when he reaches full term.

Caring for Multiples

Caring for more than one baby in the NICU brings even more challenges. Each baby will have special needs and may act in different ways than his siblings. With twins or triplets, it is especially important to ask for help from family, friends, and the NICU staff. This will allow you to spend precious time with each of your babies—getting to know them and learning how to take care of them.

Caring for Multiples in the NICU

To be sure that you get all the support you need for each baby, talk with the NICU staff about

- Placing the babies close to one another in the NICU
- Treating the babies as individuals rather than as a group, including keeping separate notes for each baby and, ideally, calling each by their first name instead of "baby A," "baby B," or "baby C"
- Color-coding incubators, bottles, and other equipment and supplies for each baby
- Finding a lactation consultant who has worked with mothers of multiples
- Finding support when you cannot be in the NICU because of work, other children at home, or needed recovery time
- Finding a support group for families with multiples

When One of Your Babies Has Gone Home but One or More Remain in the NICU

Having one or more babies in the hospital while others are at home can be very sad and difficult for new parents. Some parents feel guilty for leaving their babies at home to spend time with the babies still at the hospital, or they may feel bad for leaving the hospital to spend time with the babies at home.

All these feelings are normal. Remember that you are doing everything you can to be with all of your babies. In time, your babies will all be home and it will be easier to spend time together as a family. Check with the NICU staff to see if you are allowed to bring your other babies with you when you visit, and check with your baby's doctor to see if it is safe for your baby at home to return to a hospital environment for these visits.

Photographing Your Baby in the NICU

Many parents are reluctant to take a picture of their sick or fragile baby, but most appreciate the fact that they did, especially when they see their baby's growth and progress. Because of the special needs and environment of a baby in the NICU, here are some tips (developed by a professional photographer and mother of a former 27-weeks' gestation baby) for photographing your baby. We hope you will find it helpful to celebrate your baby's arrival and time in the NICU by taking photos, keeping journals, creating scrapbooks, or gathering other memories during this special journey.

Tip ❶: Turn off the flash.

Whether you are using a digital, disposable, or film camera, try to use natural light. The flash can scare a baby and interrupt the dark, quiet environment of the NICU. Soft window light is best, so take advantage of any windows in your baby's room. If you are taking pictures when it's dark, the overhead lights should be enough. If your baby is having phototherapy, the "bili" lights also will be enough.

Tip ❷: Step back or get close.

One unfortunate drawback to disposable cameras is that you cannot focus them, and pictures can easily get blurry. If you are using a camera that does not allow focusing, take a few steps back so your photos are sharp. You can always crop them later.

On the flip side, if you have a camera that allows you to focus, don't be afraid to get close. Close-ups of your baby's face, feet, and hands are precious. You often can work around tubes, monitors, and other hospital equipment, although, in some instances, you might want to include these to remember how things were.

Tip ❸: Think in black and white.

Consider buying some black-and-white film, or, if you have a digital camera, convert your color photos into black and white. These photographs often have a more timeless quality to them. They also soften the image by downplaying the red skin, shiny equipment, and other items near your baby.

Tip ❹: Put your baby in context.

There always comes a time when parents cannot believe their baby was ever that small. When you photograph your baby, place an item nearby that puts his small size into context, like a wedding ring or your hand. (Remember to remove all items after photographing.) That way, you'll be able to see just how small your baby was. You can remind your child of that down the road ("I remember when I could slide Daddy's wedding ring up your arm").

Tip ❺: Photograph special occasions you might want to remember.

Having a baby in the NICU doesn't mean that you cannot celebrate milestones just like you would for a full-term baby. However, NICU milestones can be very different. So remember to take pictures when

- Your baby is born (initial day[s] in the NICU).

- Your baby is weaned off the ventilator and moves to continuous positive airway pressure (CPAP), which is delivered with a scuba-like mask or nasal prongs that keep air sacs open and help your baby breathe (see *Chapter 7, Glossary of NICU Terms*).

- Your baby doesn't have any tape on his face.

- Your baby breastfeeds, tube-feeds, or bottle-feeds for the first time.

- You practice skin-to-skin (kangaroo) care with your baby for the first time.

- A sibling comes to visit for the first time.

- Your baby gets his first bath.

- Your baby moves from an incubator to a crib.

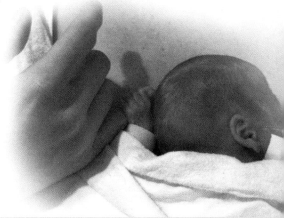

Tip ⑥: Don't forget your baby's caregivers.

The doctors and nurses in the NICU are committed to providing the best medical care for your baby. They also play an important role in caring for your family, and they form attachments to you and your baby. Take photos of your baby with special caregivers (such as doctors, nurses, therapists, and social workers). All these caring individuals are a big part of your baby's first "friends" and parent support system while your baby is in the NICU.

Tip ⑦: Share those photos.

Friends and family are not always sure how to relate to a family with a baby in the NICU. By sharing photos and updates by e-mail or in person, you can provide more information about your baby and, possibly, ease their concerns. Once you leave the NICU, the staff loves to get updates and photos of NICU "graduates," so keep the photos coming! There are several secure Web sites that allow you to share your photos with your family and friends. One example is called CaringBridge (www.caringbridge.org).

Tip ⑧: Don't expect perfection in your photos.

For many parents, it is just too overwhelming to take photos during this stressful time. If you like, leave a camera at your baby's bedside. Ask the nurses to take some photos until you feel up to the task. And don't be disappointed if your photos aren't perfect; you will still look back on them and they will stir up memories (good and bad).

While it is hard to believe right now, you will one day look back on these NICU photos and see just how far your baby has come. That is the greatest reward of all.

Siblings

The addition of a new baby to a family can be a joyful and stressful time—even more stressful when a baby needs to spend time in the NICU. If you have other children, they are part of the journey from the NICU to bringing baby home. Remember that they will need your support and help.

Here are tips adapted from the American Academy of Pediatrics (AAP) parent manual, *Understanding the NICU: What Parents of Preemies and Other Hospitalized Newborns Need to Know.*

How You Can Support Your Other Children When Your Baby Is in the NICU

- Remember to take time out for your other children. They need to know that you will continue to care for them.

- Try to answer your children's questions based on their age and what they can understand.

- Be honest and answer questions as simply as you can.

- Share pictures with younger children to help them see the baby as a real person.

- Reassure younger children that the baby's illness is not their fault.

- Help children feel important and involved. Let them pick out a special gift. Ask the NICU staff about the policies for sibling visitation.

- Understand that toddlers and preschoolers may have a hard time understanding what is happening and may even say things like, "I hate that baby!"

- Join sibling support classes.

How You Can Support Your Other Children When Your Baby Is Home From the NICU

- Remember to spend special time alone with each child.

- Understand that they may be jealous or angry when your attention is focused on caring for the special needs of their brother or sister. Children may act out to get your attention or have trouble at school. Younger children may regress to thumb-sucking or bed-wetting.

- Encourage siblings to help out if they are able to, even though it may sometimes mean more work for you.

Chapter
2
Journaling

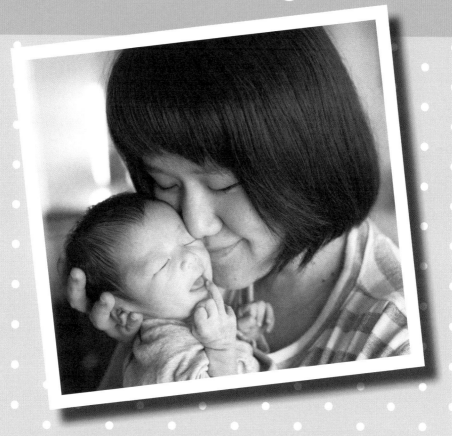

Birth Experience

A Place for Mothers to Record Memories of the Birth Experience

The date I checked in was _____

You were born on _____ at _____ am/pm.

Your actual due date was _____

The hospital where you were born was _____

The doctor who delivered you was _____

The neonatologist who took care of you was _____

About the birth: _____

_____

_____

_____

_____

_____

_____

_____

_____

_____

_____

_____

Baby's Arrival

A Place to Record Memories of Your Baby's Arrival

Your weight was _____ and your length was _____

Your eyes were _____ and your hair was _____

Your doctor first said these words about you: _____

_____

_____

Your stay in the NICU began on _____

The name we chose for you: _____

Special meaning of your name: _____

_____

Thoughts and first impressions of you: _____

_____

_____

_____

_____

_____

_____

_____

Preterm Baby Gifts

During their first weeks or months after birth, preterm babies continue to develop as if they were in their mother's womb. Because of this, preterm babies have special early growth experiences. Take time to celebrate these experiences as gifts that only preterm babies have.

Sounds

Beginning at 33 weeks' gestation, babies make a sweet noise, similar to the sound a little lamb makes. This special sound usually lasts about 5 or 6 weeks. Record your memories below.

Ears

At first, your baby's ears will lie close to his head. As he gets closer to his actual due date (around when we expected the birth to occur), the ears begin to extend and grow. Record your memories below.

Fingernails

At first, your baby might have tiny fingernails—or even just nail beds. During the first few weeks, watch closely as the nails begin to grow. Write your memories below.

Eyelashes

A baby's eyelashes may take a few weeks to grow. As you begin to see your baby's eyelashes, take time to remember this special gift below.

Footprints/Handprints

Each baby's handprints and footprints are beautiful. Each month leading up to your baby's actual due date, more lines will fill in the handprints and footprints. You may wish to ask a nurse to help take an imprint of your baby's handprints and footprints below.

Special Moments

During your baby's stay in the NICU, you will celebrate "firsts" and share many special experiences. Record these memories here so you can always recall these joyful moments.

The first time...

I saw you up close: _____

I felt your skin: _____

You began to suck: _____

You wrapped your little fingers around mine: _____

We spent time together as a family: _____

You opened your eyes: _____

We did skin-to-skin (kangaroo) care: _____

You breathed on your own: _____

I held you in my arms: _____

You looked at me: _____

I saw you without equipment: _____

You cried out loud: _____

I fed you: _____

You had a bath: _____

I bathed you: _____

You wore clothes: _____

You moved to an open crib: _____

Other special moments in the NICU: _____

Week-by-Week Memories

Keep track of milestones, medicines, procedures, and other important memories on the journal pages in this section.

Your Baby at _____ Weeks

Today's date is _____ and you are _____ weeks old.

You weigh _____ grams (_____ lb _____ oz) and you are _____ inches long.

Milestones you met this week:

_____

_____

_____

_____

How we helped take care of you this week:

_____

_____

_____

_____

Things we learned about you:

_____

_____

_____

_____

Medicines you are taking:

_____   _____

_____   _____

_____   _____

Procedures and surgeries you had this week and the follow-up care you will need:

_____

_____

_____

_____

Names of the doctors, nurses, and others who helped you:

_____   _____

_____   _____

_____   _____

Questions for the doctors, nurses, and others caring for you:

_____

_____

_____

_____

Special thoughts and memories:

_____

_____

_____

_____

_____

_____

_____

Your Baby at _____ Weeks

Today's date is _____ and you are _____ weeks old.

You weigh _____ grams (_____ lb _____ oz) and you are _____ inches long.

Milestones you met this week:

_____

_____

_____

_____

How we helped take care of you this week:

_____

_____

_____

_____

Things we learned about you:

_____

_____

_____

_____

Medicines you are taking:

_____   _____

_____   _____

_____   _____

Procedures and surgeries you had this week and the follow-up care you will need:

_____

_____

_____

_____

Names of the doctors, nurses, and others who helped you:

_____   _____

_____   _____

_____   _____

Questions for the doctors, nurses, and others caring for you:

_____

_____

_____

_____

Special thoughts and memories:

_____

_____

_____

_____

_____

_____

Your Baby at _____ Weeks

Today's date is _____ and you are _____ weeks old.

You weigh _____ grams (_____ lb _____ oz) and you are _____ inches long.

Milestones you met this week:

_____

_____

_____

_____

How we helped take care of you this week:

_____

_____

_____

_____

Things we learned about you:

_____

_____

_____

_____

Medicines you are taking:

_____   _____

_____   _____

_____   _____

Procedures and surgeries you had this week and the follow-up care you will need:

_____

_____

_____

_____

Names of the doctors, nurses, and others who helped you:

_____   _____

_____   _____

_____   _____

Questions for the doctors, nurses, and others caring for you:

_____

_____

_____

_____

Special thoughts and memories:

_____

_____

_____

_____

_____

_____

Your Baby at _____ Weeks

Today's date is _____ and you are _____ weeks old.

You weigh _____ grams (_____ lb _____ oz) and you are _____ inches long.

Milestones you met this week:

_____

_____

_____

_____

How we helped take care of you this week:

_____

_____

_____

_____

Things we learned about you:

_____

_____

_____

_____

Medicines you are taking:

_____   _____

_____   _____

_____   _____

Procedures and surgeries you had this week and the follow-up care you will need:

_____

_____

_____

Names of the doctors, nurses, and others who helped you:

_____   _____

_____   _____

_____   _____

Questions for the doctors, nurses, and others caring for you:

_____

_____

_____

Special thoughts and memories:

_____

_____

_____

_____

_____

_____

Your Baby at _____ Weeks

Today's date is _____ and you are _____ weeks old.

You weigh _____ grams (_____ lb _____ oz) and you are _____ inches long.

Milestones you met this week:

_____

_____

_____

_____

How we helped take care of you this week:

_____

_____

_____

_____

Things we learned about you:

_____

_____

_____

_____

Medicines you are taking:

_____   _____

_____   _____

_____   _____

Procedures and surgeries you had this week and the follow-up care you will need:

_____

_____

_____

_____

Names of the doctors, nurses, and others who helped you:

_____   _____

_____   _____

_____   _____

Questions for the doctors, nurses, and others caring for you:

_____

_____

_____

_____

Special thoughts and memories:

_____

_____

_____

_____

_____

_____

Your Baby at _____ Weeks

Today's date is _____ and you are _____ weeks old.

You weigh _____ grams (_____ lb _____ oz) and you are _____ inches long.

Milestones you met this week:

_____

_____

_____

_____

How we helped take care of you this week:

_____

_____

_____

_____

Things we learned about you:

_____

_____

_____

_____

Medicines you are taking:

_____   _____

_____   _____

_____   _____

Procedures and surgeries you had this week and the follow-up care you will need:

_____

_____

_____

_____

Names of the doctors, nurses, and others who helped you:

_____   _____

_____   _____

_____   _____

Questions for the doctors, nurses, and others caring for you:

_____

_____

_____

_____

Special thoughts and memories:

_____

_____

_____

_____

_____

_____

Your Baby at _____ Weeks

Today's date is _____ and you are _____ weeks old.

You weigh _____ grams (_____ lb _____ oz) and you are _____ inches long.

Milestones you met this week:

_____

_____

_____

_____

How we helped take care of you this week:

_____

_____

_____

_____

Things we learned about you:

_____

_____

_____

_____

Medicines you are taking:

_____   _____

_____   _____

_____   _____

Procedures and surgeries you had this week and the follow-up care you will need:

_____

_____

_____

_____

Names of the doctors, nurses, and others who helped you:

_____   _____

_____   _____

_____   _____

Questions for the doctors, nurses, and others caring for you:

_____

_____

_____

_____

Special thoughts and memories:

_____

_____

_____

_____

_____

_____

Your Baby at _____ Weeks

Today's date is _____ and you are _____ weeks old.

You weigh _____ grams (_____ lb _____ oz) and you are _____ inches long.

Milestones you met this week:

_____

_____

_____

_____

How we helped take care of you this week:

_____

_____

_____

_____

Things we learned about you:

_____

_____

_____

_____

Medicines you are taking:

_____   _____

_____   _____

_____   _____

Procedures and surgeries you had this week and the follow-up care you will need:

_____

_____

_____

_____

Names of the doctors, nurses, and others who helped you:

_____   _____

_____   _____

_____   _____

Questions for the doctors, nurses, and others caring for you:

_____

_____

_____

_____

Special thoughts and memories:

_____

_____

_____

_____

_____

_____

_____

Your Baby at _____ Weeks

Today's date is _____ and you are _____ weeks old.

You weigh _____ grams (_____ lb _____ oz) and you are _____ inches long.

Milestones you met this week:

_____

_____

_____

_____

How we helped take care of you this week:

_____

_____

_____

_____

Things we learned about you:

_____

_____

_____

_____

Medicines you are taking:

_____   _____

_____   _____

_____   _____

Procedures and surgeries you had this week and the follow-up care you will need:

_____

_____

_____

_____

Names of the doctors, nurses, and others who helped you:

_____   _____

_____   _____

_____   _____

Questions for the doctors, nurses, and others caring for you:

_____

_____

_____

_____

Special thoughts and memories:

_____

_____

_____

_____

_____

_____

Your Baby at _____ Weeks

Today's date is _____ and you are _____ weeks old.

You weigh _____ grams (_____ lb _____ oz) and you are _____ inches long.

Milestones you met this week:

_____

_____

_____

_____

How we helped take care of you this week:

_____

_____

_____

_____

Things we learned about you:

_____

_____

_____

_____

Medicines you are taking:

_____   _____

_____   _____

_____   _____

Procedures and surgeries you had this week and the follow-up care you will need:

_____

_____

_____

_____

Names of the doctors, nurses, and others who helped you:

_____   _____

_____   _____

_____   _____

Questions for the doctors, nurses, and others caring for you:

_____

_____

_____

_____

Special thoughts and memories:

_____

_____

_____

_____

_____

_____

Chapter
3
Taking Care of You

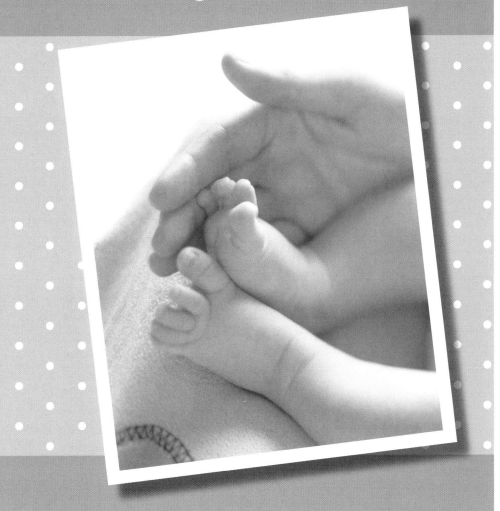

Coping

Having a baby in a NICU is very stressful for parents. The uncertainty, the highs and lows, and the decisions all take their toll.

If, at first, you feel distant from your baby, you may wonder if there is something wrong with you, or you may worry that because you cannot snuggle with your baby, you won't be able to bond. Rest assured that feeling distant is a normal reaction for parents during the early weeks of their baby's NICU stay. Feeling distant doesn't mean you are not bonding. Your bond with your baby began during pregnancy and continues to grow long after your baby is born. Be patient with yourself. Over time, as you adjust to the NICU, you'll feel closer and more like a parent to your baby.

As time passes and your emotions change, keep in mind that most parents of babies in the NICU feel many positive and negative feelings—even at the same time. This is because your heartfelt connection with your baby includes joy and pain.

The NICU Roller Coaster

For many families, the NICU stay is like a roller coaster ride, with ups and downs, triumphs and setbacks. The following tips may help you deal with your ups and downs:

- Give yourself permission to cry and feel overwhelmed. You may worry that you'll never be able to pull yourself back together, but you will.

- Get into a routine. Find a way to balance work, home, and visiting the hospital. Allow yourself to leave your baby's side when you can. While your baby needs you, it is also important to have time to yourself, with your partner, and with your other children. Also take time to do things you enjoy, like exercise. These restful breaks will help you find the strength to keep going.

- Connect with other parents of babies in the NICU. They share many of your feelings and struggles. Talk together, informally or in a support group. Ask the NICU staff if there are parents of babies who have graduated from the NICU with whom you can connect for support, or if there are other community resources.

- Explore your spiritual side. It might be helpful to reflect and lean on your spiritual beliefs. You may find comfort talking with a pastor, priest, rabbi, minister, or imam. It is normal for this experience to challenge your religious and spiritual beliefs. However, prayer, meditation, or quiet reflection can help you find emotional strength and hope during this challenging time.

- Keep a journal. Expressing your feelings on paper can help you cope with your emotional changes. A journal also strengthens your hope and patience by reminding you how far you and your baby have come.

- Vent your frustrations. If your baby has a setback, you may be plunged back into fear and anxiety. Voice your fears, and hope for the best.

- Celebrate when you can. When your baby makes progress, it is OK to experience the joy.

- Accept the support of others, however clumsy it may seem. Let people know how they can best help you.

- Accept that you and your partner will react differently. Share your experiences and listen with empathy so that you each can feel supported.

You and Your Partner

During your baby's NICU stay, your partner can be your greatest source of support, but there may be times when you find it difficult to deal with each other. It's only natural that your reactions will be as unique as you are. The painful feelings so common to the NICU experience can add stress to your relationship. The following tips may help you weather the crisis together:

- Share your thoughts, feelings, information, and burdensome tasks with each other. Lean on each other's strengths and forgive weaknesses. Remember that you both want what is best for your baby.

- Manage conflict with listening, compromise, and respect.

- Empathize with each other. When your partner is venting, don't try to fix it. Just listen and understand. Supporting each other is the best comfort.

- Make time to kindle and nurture your relationship, so that you can turn to it for strength.

- Learn about the signs of post-traumatic stress disorder. Get professional help if needed.

Parents Without Partners in the NICU

If you are separated, divorced, single, or widowed, you may feel very alone without a partner to share the burdens and joys. You may find it difficult to be the only one handling all the information and decisions. Being a single parent, you play a role that is challenging but very important.

All parents need support. When you don't have a partner, it is natural to confide in a trusted family member or friend about your fears and concerns. Reach out to those close to you for the help you need. A NICU parent support group or other parents of babies in the NICU also can provide you with much-needed comfort and partnership.

The March of Dimes online community for NICU families, Share Your Story (www.shareyourstory.org), offers support and information for families of babies in the NICU or who are home from the NICU. You can join in discussion with others who have very similar experiences to yours, ask questions, get support, participate in live online chats, and even offer your story and support to others.

Postpartum Depression

As a new mother, it is normal to have many intense feelings, especially while your baby is in the NICU. It is not uncommon for new mothers to find that they may react differently or more passionately to some things than they may have prior to giving birth. This is completely normal. When do you know if what you are experiencing is something more than what would be expected for this time in your life? If you are having trouble dealing with the intense feelings, you may have some level of postpartum depression.

How do I know if I have postpartum depression?

If you have any of the following feelings and cannot get rid of them, you may have postpartum depression:

- Sadness.
- Tiredness.
- Anger.
- Loss of hope.
- Loss of interest in things you like.
- Your ability to cope is not improving and you feel stuck.
- You find no joy in other parts of your life.
- You have trouble with your relationship with your partner or others close to you.
- You feel a parent support group isn't "quite enough."

It is essential to speak with a professional counselor if you

- Feel prolonged numbness or detachment.
- Continue to feel detached from your baby.
- Have trouble getting out of bed or starting your day.
- Feel unable to cope or manage your other responsibilities.
- Think about harming yourself or others.

A professional counselor can help. Your doctor or a hospital social worker can refer you to a counselor who understands the trauma of having a baby in the NICU. Even just a couple of visits might give you the reassurance and boost you need. Visiting a counselor and asking for help is nothing to be ashamed about; it will just help you cope better.

Content from **www.marchofdimes.org**, *March of Dimes Foundation (2009). Reprinted with permission. For more information, go to* **www.marchofdimes.org** *or* **http://nacersano.marchofdimes.org**. *To order materials, go to* **www.marchofdimes.org/catalog**. *For comfort, support, and information from others who understand the challenges and uncertainties of the NICU experience, visit the March of Dimes online community for NICU families,* **www.shareyourstory.org**.

Importance of a Smoke-free Environment

It is very important for you to provide a smoke-free environment for your baby. Babies' lungs are not completely mature at birth and take 2 to 3 years to develop all the small air sacs necessary for a lifetime of healthy lung function. Tobacco smoke irritates the airways of babies and affects the growth of their lungs during the first 2 to 3 years of their lives, when their lungs are continuing to develop.

Preterm babies are especially prone to having lung problems after discharge from the NICU. Being exposed to tobacco smoke makes these lung problems worse and makes preterm babies more prone to develop airway infections and obstruction. When their parents smoke, preterm babies smoke!

Many parents think that, as long as they smoke outside, their smoking does not harm their baby, but this is not true. Even when you smoke outside, chemicals from the tobacco smoke cling to your clothes and continue to irritate your baby's airways, causing inflammation and airway injury. Anyone who smokes around a baby or young child is harming their precious child with secondhand smoke.

Secondhand smoke exposure has been well documented in many research studies to cause harm to babies and children. Babies exposed to secondhand smoke have more upper and lower respiratory illnesses, more ear infections, an increased rate of asthma, more frequent visits to the doctor, and more hospitalizations. Babies who are exposed to cigarette smoke have twice the occurrence of sudden infant death syndrome (SIDS) and are at increased risk for behavioral problems, such as attention-deficit/hyperactivity disorder (ADHD).

The poisons from tobacco smoke cling to home furniture, drapes, carpets, ceilings, and walls, as well as car seats, for years. This is known as "thirdhand smoke" because the toxic fumes are present in the environment for months to years later. It is important that you thoroughly clean your home and car when transforming them into smoke-free environments. A smoke-free home and car are essential for your baby to breathe safely.

Chemicals from tobacco smoke contaminate the breast milk that mothers produce. Breastfeeding is important for all babies to provide optimal nutrition and brain development as well as protection from infections. Because the protective benefits of breastfeeding are present even if a mother smokes, mothers who smoke are still encouraged to breastfeed their babies. If a mother who breastfeeds uses nicotine replacement therapy, this is much better for her baby than smoking. Of course, having no exposure to tobacco toxins is best for mother and baby.

Babies and children who are exposed to secondhand smoke have much more serious health problems than babies or children who are not exposed to second-hand smoke. The consequences of using tobacco products is something we wish to help you avoid for the health of you and your baby.

Please let us know if you would like help in becoming a nonsmoker or if you have any questions about providing a smoke-free home and car for your baby. For the health of your baby and your own health, it is essential that you and everyone in your household stop smoking.

Because tobacco products contain nicotine, which is very addictive, it is hard for most people to quit smoking. Fortunately, there is help, which can make it easier to quit smoking, even if you have tried quitting before without success. This time you can succeed. Ask the NICU staff for more information and call 1-800-QUIT-NOW (784-8669) for help in quitting and in making your home and car smoke free.

Chapter
4
The Journey Home

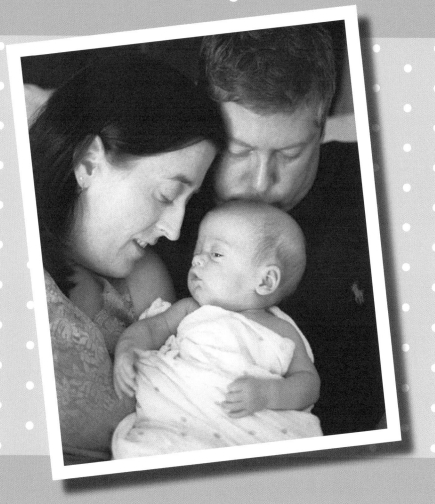

Bringing Your Baby Home From the NICU

As your baby grows stronger and healthier, the time will come to take him home. While some parents may feel excited, they also may worry about caring for their baby on their own. The NICU staff will work with families to make sure they know how to care for their baby on their own. Use the following checklists as you prepare to go home:

Preparing for Your Baby to Leave the NICU

In the Hospital

☐ Add your baby to your health insurance policy.

☐ Speak with a social worker to see if you qualify for state or local services and fill out the paperwork while your baby is still in the hospital.

☐ Request a predischarge meeting with your baby's health care team to talk about your baby's medical needs and what to expect in the months and years ahead.

☐ Choose a primary care provider, such as pediatrician, for your baby after discharge from the hospital, asking specific questions about his or her experience and any special care given for a preterm or sick baby.

☐ If your baby is going to be on Medicaid and you are going to receive aid from Women, Infants, and Children (also known as WIC), set it up while you are in the hospital.

Pediatric and Specialty Care

☐ Schedule your baby's first visit with your baby's doctor.

☐ Schedule any follow-up appointments with specialists.

☐ Ask the NICU staff if your baby qualifies for an Early Intervention evaluation and have this scheduled before leaving the hospital.

☐ Make sure your baby has received all required immunizations.

☐ File your baby's immunization record in a folder for safekeeping and for upcoming health care visits.

- [ ] If your baby was born at or before 30 weeks' gestation, make sure he has an eye examination. Ask if you need to schedule a follow-up eye examination for your baby.

- [ ] Ask for the results of your baby's hearing screening. Also, ask if you need to schedule a follow-up visit for your baby.

- [ ] Get a copy of your baby's discharge summary for your records and be sure to review any and all questions about his care up until this point from your notes in this *NICU Journal.*

- [ ] Get all your baby's prescriptions from the doctors and review them with his health care team so that you are sure you understand how and when to administer any medicines and have them filled.

- [ ] Make sure you know about respiratory syncytial virus (RSV) season and what you need to do to protect your baby during the RSV season. Some babies may qualify for monthly RSV prophylaxis. Ask your baby's doctor about this.

- [ ] Review the signs and symptoms of sickness that would make you call or visit your baby's doctor.

- [ ] Ask the NICU staff if you can stay in the NICU overnight ("room in") with your baby before discharge.

- [ ] Talk to the social worker if you are worried about electricity, phone service, transportation, or food when your baby leaves the NICU.

Safety

- [ ] Take a CPR (also known as cardiopulmonary resuscitation) class.

- [ ] Get a car seat for your baby. Sometimes, preterm babies have special needs because of their size and strength. They may need a car bed because of problems with apnea, oxygenation, or heart rate. Ask your health care team what is best for your baby.

- [ ] Bring your baby's car seat to the hospital for a car seat test.

- [ ] Ask the NICU staff when your baby can safely go out in public.

- [ ] Discuss "back to sleep" and "tummy time" with your NICU staff. See *Safe Sleep and Your Baby* later in this chapter.

Preparing for Your Baby's Medical Needs at Home

☐ Discuss with your health care team any special medical supplies you will need in your home.

☐ Learn about any equipment your baby will need at home and who to call for additional questions.

☐ Learn how to order more equipment or supplies for your baby.

Preparing Your Home for Your Baby's Arrival

Preparing your home for your baby's arrival can help keep your baby healthy and safe. To prepare your home for your baby, you can

- Gather and store baby supplies, such as diapers, blankets, washcloths, formula (if you are not breastfeeding), bottles (for breast milk or formula), and a digital (not mercury) thermometer.

- Prepare a crib for your baby or talk about other sleeping options for your baby with your baby's doctor.

- Post emergency phone numbers next to all the phones in your home.

- Clean your house of dust, pet hairs, paint smells, tobacco smoke, or other smells that may bother your baby's eyes, nose, and lungs.

- Teach everyone in your home about good hand washing. Be sure to have soap by all bathroom sinks. Having hand sanitizer in any rooms in which you will take your baby is recommended.

- Make sure household members and caregivers are immunized against whopping cough (pertussis) and influenza. Preterm babies are especially vulnerable to these infections, which can cause severe lung infections and even death in babies.

- Provide a smoke-free environment for your baby (see *Importance of a Smoke-free Environment* in Chapter 3, Taking Care of You).

- Discuss with extended family and friends the precautions you will be taking to ensure continued good health of your baby. Ask for their respect and support in doing so. Such precautions include

  - Not allowing smoking in your home.

  - Asking anyone who may be "coming down with something" to postpone his or her visit.

  - Teaching everyone to do proper hand washing prior to touching your baby.

  - Limiting the number and length of time you have guests (outside family included) and, initially, the number of small children other than those who already live with you to, ideally, reduce the possibility of exposure to illnesses, especially during cold and flu season.

  - Discussing safety of family or cultural traditions with your baby's doctor. For example, some parents want to know how soon a baby's ears can be pierced, and some cultures place "protective" strings, amulets, or jewelry on their babies after discharge.

Preparing for Your Baby's Nutritional Needs at Home

- Discuss with your health care team the special feeding needs of your baby at home.

- Take any stored breast milk home and review the care and thawing process for use at home.

- Babies who have been born prematurely may need to continue to receive additional nutrition after discharge with special formulas if they are not receiving breast milk. This is to help these babies grow and improve their health. Babies receiving breast milk may also require a supplement.

- Consult your baby's doctor about whether any supplements are needed after discharge. These special formulas or breast milk supplements, used after discharge, may contain extra protein, calcium, phosphorous, vitamins, and minerals that promote adequate growth and provide energy. Again, your baby's doctor will determine which nutritional strategy to follow when you take your baby home and how to monitor your baby's growth and development.

Transportation Needs

All 50 states have laws requiring the use of infant safety seats in the car, and it has become standard hospital policy that parents must have one in their possession before taking their new baby home. Showing up with a car safety seat, however, is not the same as using and installing it correctly. Make sure you use the installation tips provided by the manufacturer. Visit your local fire station or police station to ensure your car seat is properly installed in your car.

The "Car Seat Challenge"

For babies born more than 3 weeks prematurely, the AAP recommends that they be monitored in their car seat before leaving the hospital. Taking this simple precaution helps ensure that the car seat's semi-reclined position won't cause your baby to experience breathing problems or slowing of his heartbeat. When it is a problem, your baby's doctor may recommend that your baby use a car bed. Hospital staff who are trained in positioning babies properly in the car seat and in detecting apnea, bradycardia, and oxygen desaturation should conduct the car safety seat observation or "challenge." Ask your health care team to review the car seat observation with you and go over proper positioning for your baby.

Car safety seats ("regular" infant car seats) are recognized to provide excellent protection for babies positioned rear facing and are the preferred method of transportation. Car beds are meant for babies who cannot be safely restrained in a regular car seat and must be transported lying down. Most commonly, this applies to very small or preterm babies. Car seats and beds should never be bought secondhand or reused unless advised by a child passenger safety technician. Unlike car seats, most car beds are designed for use by a single baby only—even if only used for a few days or weeks.

The key to keeping your baby safe in the car lies not just in buying an appropriate car seat but also in using it properly. Properly installed car safety seats have been shown to dramatically reduce the number of deaths (by some estimates, >70%) in infants younger than 1 year. A guide for families on car seat safety can be found at www.HealthyChildren.org, the official AAP Web site for parents.

Early Intervention Program

Preterm babies and babies born with certain medical conditions develop at their own pace, and, along the way, they may need special Early Intervention services. Early Intervention is the official name for the extra care some children receive to help them develop, grow, and learn. An evaluation for Early Intervention services is available to your baby after discharge (anytime between birth and age 3 years) if he meets any of the following criteria:

- Your baby was admitted to the NICU or had a serious illness at birth that could affect his development.

- Your baby was born with a low birth weight of less than 2,500 g or born very preterm at less than 33 weeks' gestation.

- Your baby was born with a birth abnormality that affects his brain, muscles, or nervous system.

- Your baby was exposed to alcohol or drugs before, during, or following your pregnancy.

- Your baby has been involved in a protective services case or program.

Ask your baby's NICU staff for information on how to set up an appointment for a free evaluation. Remember, you can ask for an evaluation even if you are not worried about your baby's progress or development. Qualifications can vary among states, so ask your baby's doctor about the Early Intervention program in your state.

When Your Baby Must Transfer Hospitals or Units

Transferring Your Baby to Another NICU

If your baby is very sick, he may need to go to a larger hospital or a regional perinatal (medical) center. These hospitals often have more specialists and resources to help babies with special health care needs. If your baby is moving to another hospital, talk with the NICU staff about how this will happen. Usually, your baby's current doctor will coordinate with the new NICU to help prepare your baby for traveling.

It may not be possible for you to travel with your baby. Ask the NICU staff about this. Make sure that you have the contact information for the new NICU so you can call to check on your baby at any time.

Transferring Your Baby to an Intermediate Care Nursery

Very ill babies are cared for in the NICU. As they begin to recover, they often go to an intermediate care nursery. This may be another unit in the same hospital or at a different hospital.

The intermediate care nursery staff are trained to give the special medical attention babies need to grow stronger and more stable. If your baby is moving to an intermediate care nursery, talk with your baby's doctor about how you can prepare for the change. For example, you may want to visit the new nursery and talk with the staff before your baby is transferred.

Immunization and Medical Records

Before discharge, your baby will receive

- Immunizations

- An eye examination (if needed)

- A hearing screening

- Newborn screening blood spot tests (also known as the heel prick test)

- Critical congenital heart disease screening

- Head sonogram if born before 32 weeks' gestation

- Several doses of important medicines (if needed)

Keep a record of when your baby gets each of these and note any follow-up you will need to do (when, where, and with whom, as well as the contact information, address, and directions to the office). Learn more about common NICU tests on the March of Dimes Web site at **www.marchofdimes.org/complications/ common-nicu-tests.aspx**.

Immunizations

Immunizations protect your baby from many infections. This section includes a list of the ones your baby needs and a place for you to keep track of when your baby gets them. Preterm babies get their immunizations at the same age as full-term babies, except for the initial dose of hepatitis B vaccine. Generally, no correction is made for being born early, and vaccinations are not delayed. It is very important that parents of preterm babies, as well as those of all babies, adhere to the recommended schedule for these immunizations. Some of these diseases have resurged in recent years in the United States, and babies who have been in the NICU are at increased risk for complications if they were exposed to them. It is equally important that parents, siblings, and all caregivers are also immunized against whooping cough (pertussis) and influenza. Preterm babies are especially vulnerable to these infections, which can cause severe lung infections and even death in young babies.

Hepatitis B

Hepatitis B is a serious disease that affects the liver. Hepatitis B vaccine prevents hepatitis B virus infection and its serious consequences, including liver cancer and cirrhosis. Three doses of the hepatitis B vaccine are safe and highly effective. The first shot is usually given after birth but before discharge from the hospital to full-term babies. The second shot is given between 1 and 4 months of age. The third shot is given between 6 and 18 months of age. If your baby is preterm, the timing of the doses may vary and your child may need more than 3 doses of the vaccine. Your baby's doctor will tell you when shots will be given.

You were given the hepatitis B vaccine on the following dates:

First dose: _____

Second dose: _____

Third dose: _____

Fourth dose (if needed): _____

Follow-up needed after discharge: _____

_____

_____

Diphtheria, Tetanus, and Acellular Pertussis

The diphtheria, tetanus, and acellular pertussis (DTaP) vaccine helps protect your baby from 3 diseases: diphtheria, tetanus, and pertussis (whooping cough). Three shots of the vaccine are needed within the first year after birth. A fourth shot is given at 15 through 18 months. The fifth shot will be given at 4 through 6 years.

You were given the DTaP vaccine on the following dates:

First dose: _____

Second dose: _____

Third dose: _____

Fourth dose: _____

Fifth dose: _____

Follow-up needed after discharge: _____

_____

_____

Haemophilus influenzae *type b*

Haemophilus influenzae type b (Hib) is a type of bacteria that can cause several kinds of serious infections, including meningitis. Two or 3 shots of the Hib vaccine are needed within your baby's first 6 months after birth. A booster dose is given at 12 to 15 months.

You were given the Hib vaccine on the following dates:

First dose: _____

Second dose: _____

Third dose: _____

Booster: _____

Follow-up needed after discharge: _____

_____

_____

Polio

Three shots of the polio vaccine (also called inactivated poliovirus vaccine, or IPV) are given between 2 and 18 months of age. A booster shot will be given when your child is between 4 and 6 years of age.

You were given the polio vaccine on the following dates:

First dose: _____

Second dose: _____

Third dose: _____

Booster: _____

Follow-up needed after discharge: _____

_____

Measles, Mumps, and Rubella

The measles, mumps, and rubella (MMR) vaccine will help protect your baby from measles, mumps, and rubella (German measles). The first shot is given when your child is between 12 and 15 months old. A second shot is usually given when your child is between 4 and 6 years of age but can be administered as early as 28 days after the first dose.

You were given the MMR vaccine on the following dates:

First dose: _____

Second dose: _____

Follow-up needed after discharge: _____

_____

_____

Pneumococcal

Pneumococcus is a type of bacteria that can attack different parts of the body and cause serious infections. Three doses of this vaccine are given when your baby is 2, 4, and 6 months old. A fourth dose is given when your baby is between 12 and 15 months of age. If your baby is late getting these shots, check with your baby's doctor to see if fewer shots are needed and when your baby should get them.

You were given the pneumococcal vaccine on the following dates:

First dose: _____

Second dose: _____

Third dose: _____

Fourth dose: _____

Follow-up needed after discharge: _____

_____

Influenza (Flu)

The influenza (flu) vaccine is given each year to all infants, children, and adolescents between 6 months and 18 years of age. It is very important that, if your baby is younger than 6 months, all family members and caregivers get the flu vaccine to protect your baby from catching the flu. Influenza infections in preterm babies cause them to become critically ill. The first year that your baby receives the flu vaccine, he will get 2 shots separated by 4 weeks.

You were given the flu vaccine on the following dates:

First dose: _____

Second dose (4 weeks after first dose): _____

Follow-up needed after discharge: _____

_____

Varicella (Chickenpox)

One dose of the varicella (commonly known as chickenpox) vaccine is given when your child is between 12 and 15 months old. A second shot is given when your child is 4 to 6 years of age, but it can be administered earlier.

You were given the varicella (chickenpox) vaccine on the following dates:

First dose: _____

Second dose: _____

Follow-up needed after discharge: _____

_____

Other Immunizations

If your baby's doctor recommends other vaccines for your baby, record the dates your baby received the doses.

You were given the _____ **vaccine on the following dates:**

First dose: _____

Second dose: _____

Third dose: _____

Follow-up needed after discharge: _____

_____

You were given the _____ vaccine on the following dates:

First dose: _____

Second dose: _____

Third dose: _____

Follow-up needed after discharge: _____

_____

_____

Combination Vaccines

Your baby's doctor may combine vaccines to reduce the number of shots your baby needs to receive to stay healthy. If you are interested in combining your baby's vaccines, check with your baby's doctor to see if any are available.

Examples of common combination vaccines include

- DTaP and Hib vaccine
- Hib and hepatitis B vaccine
- DTaP, hepatitis B, and polio vaccine
- MMR and varicella (chickenpox) vaccine

Note: Immunization information is updated periodically. Please go to **www.HealthyChildren.org** *for the most current information.*

Respiratory Syncytial Virus: More Than a Cold

Respiratory syncytial virus, or RSV, is a very common illness in infancy and early childhood. Most infants get RSV during their first year after birth, and almost all children are infected by the time they are 2 years old. For most healthy children, RSV is like a cold. However, for some preterm babies and for those with certain types of lung or heart problems, it can be dangerous. This is because preterm babies, even those who did not need any additional help breathing while they were in the NICU, do not have fully developed lungs. Also, they may not have received virus-fighting substances (called *antibodies*) to help fight off RSV and other viruses. It is common for parents to feel that their once very tiny and fragile baby now appears very healthy and robust, but it is still extremely important during the first year after birth to take specific precautions to decrease exposure to RSV, if at all possible. If your baby is younger than 1 year at the beginning of RSV season, you should take appropriate precautions, such as continued proper hand washing and limiting exposure to crowds and school-aged children. Some babies may need monthly RSV vaccinations during the RSV season. Ask your baby's doctor for additional suggestions.

Respiratory syncytial virus infections tend to occur at a certain time of the year. The season usually starts in the fall and ends in the spring. Talk with your baby's doctor about the RSV season in your area. For babies born before 29 weeks' gestation or with certain other risk factors, you need to take special precautions to help ensure they are not exposed to a person with RSV or any other cold or flu virus. It is also very important to be sure your child is not exposed to secondhand smoke. Breastfeeding will help protect your baby from many types of infection.

Respiratory syncytial virus is contagious. It can be spread through the air when a person coughs or sneezes. It also can spread by touching an object that has the virus on it. In fact, the virus can live on countertops, doorknobs, hands, and clothing for up to 7 hours. Hand washing and proper cleaning are the best ways to help prevent the spread of RSV.

Symptoms of RSV

Respiratory syncytial virus usually causes a mild cold with a runny nose and fever. However, in some babies, the symptoms can become severe. Call your baby's doctor right away if your baby has any of the following symptoms:

- Cough that does not go away or gets worse
- Wheezing (a high-pitched whistling sound when breathing)
- Trouble breathing or breathing faster than usual
- Blue color on the lips or around the mouth
- High fever
- Thick nasal discharge

Eye and Ear Health

A baby's eye and ear health is very important, especially when he was born prematurely. When your baby gets his eye examination and hearing screening, you can keep track of the results and the necessary follow-up care with a hearing or vision specialist.

You had your newborn eye examination on this date: _____

Results: _____

_____

Follow-up needed after discharge: _____

_____

You had your newborn hearing screening on this date: _____

Left ear   Right ear

☐ Passed   ☐ Failed   ☐ Passed   ☐ Failed

Follow-up needed after discharge: _____

_____

Safe Sleep and Your Baby

About 3,500 babies die each year in the United States during sleep because of unsafe sleep environments. Some of these deaths are from entrapment, suffocation, and strangulation. Some babies die from SIDS, which is the sudden, unexplained death of a baby younger than 1 year. Here are ways for you to keep your sleeping baby safe.

Note: These recommendations are for healthy babies up to 1 year of age. A very small number of babies with certain medical conditions may need to be placed to sleep on their stomachs. Your baby's doctor can tell you what is best for your baby.

- Place your baby to sleep on his back for every sleep until he is 1 year old. If your baby has rolled onto his side or stomach, he can be left in that position if he is already able to roll from tummy to back and back to tummy. If your baby falls asleep in a car safety seat, stroller, swing, infant carrier, or infant sling, he should be moved to a firm sleep surface as soon as possible.

- Place your baby to sleep on a firm sleep surface. The crib, bassinet, portable crib, or play yard should meet current safety standards. Do not put blankets or pillows between the mattress and the fitted sheet. Never put your baby to sleep on a chair, sofa, waterbed, cushion, or sheepskin.

- Keep soft objects, loose bedding, or any objects that could increase the risk of entrapment, suffocation, or strangulation out of the crib. These objects include pillows, quilts, comforters, sheepskins, bumper pads, and stuffed toys. *Note:* Research has not shown us when it's 100% safe to have these objects in the crib; however, most experts agree that after 12 months of age these objects pose little health risk to healthy babies.

- Place your baby to sleep in the same room where you sleep but not the same bed. This is the safest sleep arrangement for your baby. Put your baby's crib close to your bed so that you can easily watch and feed your baby.

- Breastfeed as much and for as long as you can.

- Make sure that your baby gets all recommended immunizations.

- Keep your baby away from smokers and places where people smoke.

- Do not let your baby get too hot. Keep the room where your baby sleeps at a comfortable temperature. In general, dress your baby in no more than one extra layer than you would wear. Your baby may be too hot if he is sweating or if his chest feels hot. If you are worried that your baby is cold, use a wearable blanket, such as a sleeping sack, or warm sleeper that is the right size for your baby. These are made to cover the body and not the head.

- Offer a pacifier at nap time and bedtime. This helps to reduce the risk of SIDS. If you are breastfeeding, wait until breastfeeding is going well before offering a pacifier. It's OK if your baby doesn't want to use a pacifier. If the baby's pacifier falls out after he falls asleep, you don't have to put it back in.

Chapter
5
Supporting You and Your Baby: Milestone Guidelines

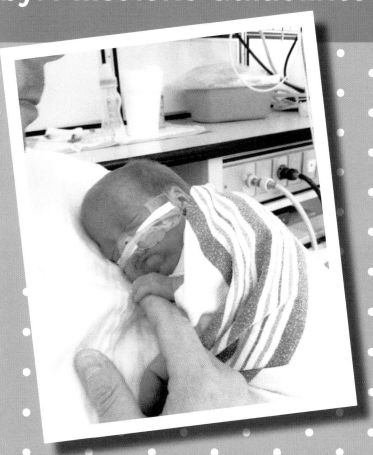

Having a baby—whether it's your first child or your fourth—is so exciting! But it is not always easy. If your baby was born more than 3 weeks early, you may have more questions about your baby and how he will grow than a parent whose baby was born on time.

We wrote this section to help you understand how your baby will develop. We have listed important *milestones,* or achievements, in a baby's growth, so you know what to watch for at each age. For example, typical milestones for babies are, "Makes eye contact and smiles," and "Rolls over from tummy to back."

It is important to remember that development is not a race. Babies develop at their own speed and in their own way. Some babies do not reach every milestone at the same time. *This is especially true if they were born early.*

Adjusted Age

Keep in mind that babies develop at their own speed and in their own way. However, parents of preterm babies will need to adjust their baby's age to get a true sense of where their baby should be in his development.

Here's what to do.
Subtract the number of weeks your baby was born early from your baby's actual age in weeks (number of weeks since the date of birth). This is your baby's *adjusted age* (also called *corrected age*).

Examples of Adjusted Ages

Actual Age	Weeks Born Early	Adjusted Age
8 weeks (2 months)	3 weeks	5 weeks (1 month and 1 week)
16 weeks (4 months)	4 weeks	12 weeks (3 months)
24 weeks (6 months)	5 weeks	19 weeks (4 months and 3 weeks)

Calculate your baby's adjusted age.

_____ – _____ = _____

       Actual age   Weeks born early   Adjusted age

NOTE: The number of months is based on a 4-week month. Also, by 2 years of age, most children have caught up to the typical milestone range. If your child has not caught up, he may need extra support for a longer period.

Your Child's Progress

You know your child better than anyone else. Even with an adjusted age, you will want to see him move forward in his development. For example, your child should progress from pulling himself up, to standing, and then to walking. When you watch him carefully, you will see ways he is growing well. You will also know whether he needs more help. Remember to take your child to his recommended well-child (health supervision) visits. At each visit, your child's doctor will check his progress and ask you about the ways you see your child growing. See the next section, Developmental Milestones.

Developmental Milestones

Here is information about how babies and young children typically develop. Examples of developmental milestones for ages 1 month to 6 years are listed. The developmental milestones are listed by month or year first because well-child visits are organized this way.

For a preterm baby, it is important to use the baby's adjusted age when tracking development until 2 years of age so that his growth and progress take into account that he was born early.

What is your child's adjusted age? _____. See milestone for the adjusted age in the next section.

NOTE: Ask your baby's doctor about Early Intervention (EI)—extra care some babies and children receive to help them develop.

· · · · · · · · · · · · · · · · · **At 1 Month (4 Weeks)** · · · · · · · · · · · · · · · ·

Social
▸ Looks at parent; follows parent with eyes
▸ Has self-comforting behaviors, such as bringing hands to mouth
▸ Starts to become fussy when bored; calms when picked up or spoken to
▸ Looks briefly at objects

Language

- Makes brief, short vowel sounds
- Alerts to unexpected sound; quiets or turns to parent's voice
- Shows signs of sensitivity to environment (such as excessive crying, tremors, or excessive startles) or need for extra support to handle activities of daily living
- Has different types of cries for hunger and tiredness

Motor

- Moves both arms and both legs together
- Holds chin up when on tummy
- Opens fingers slightly when at rest

· · · · · · · · · · · · · · · **At 2 Months (8 Weeks)** · · · · · · · · · · · · · · · · ·

Social

- Smiles responsively
- Makes sounds that show happiness or upset

Language

- Makes short cooing sounds

Motor

- Opens and shuts hands
- Briefly brings hands together
- Lifts head and chest when lying on tummy
- Keeps head steady when held in a sitting position

· · · · · · · · · · · · · · · **At 4 Months (16 Weeks)** · · · · · · · · · · · · · · · · ·

Social

- Laughs aloud
- Looks for parent or another caregiver when upset

Language

- Turns to voices
- Makes long cooing sounds

Motor
- Supports self on elbows and wrists when on tummy
- Rolls over from tummy to back
- Keeps hands unfisted
- Plays with fingers near middle of body
- Grasps objects

························ **At 6 Months (24 Weeks)** ····················

Social
- Pats or smiles at own reflection
- Looks when name is called

Language
- Babbles, making sounds such as "da," "ga," "ba," or "ka"

Motor
- Sits briefly without support
- Rolls over from back to tummy
- Passes a toy from one hand to another
- Rakes small objects with 4 fingers to pick them up
- Bangs small objects on surface

························ **At 9 Months (36 Weeks)** ····················

Social
- Uses basic gestures (such as holding out arms to be picked up or waving bye-bye)
- Looks for dropped objects
- Plays games such as peekaboo and pat-a-cake
- Turns consistently when name called

Language
- Says "Dada" or "Mama" nonspecifically
- Looks around when hearing things such as "Where's your bottle?" or "Where's your blanket?"
- Copies sounds that parent or caregiver makes

Motor

- Sits well without support
- Pulls to stand
- Moves easily between sitting and lying
- Crawls on hands and knees
- Picks up food to eat
- Picks up small objects with 3 fingers and thumb
- Lets go of objects on purpose
- Bangs objects together

•••••••••••• **At 12 Months (48 Weeks, or 1 Year)** ••••••••••••

Social

- Looks for hidden objects
- Imitates new gestures

Language

- Uses "Dada" or "Mama" specifically
- Uses 1 word other than *Mama, Dada,* or a personal name
- Follows directions with gestures, such as motioning and saying, "Give me (object)."

Motor

- Takes first steps
- Stands without support
- Drops an object into a cup
- Picks up small object with 1 finger and thumb
- Picks up food to eat

•••••••••• **At 15 Months (60 Weeks, or 1¼ Years)** ••••••••••

Social

- Imitates scribbling
- Drinks from cup with little spilling
- Points to ask something or get help
- Looks around after hearing things such as "Where's your ball?" or "Where's your blanket?"

Language
- Uses 3 words other than names
- Speaks in what sounds like an unknown language
- Follows directions that do not include a gesture

Motor
- Squats to pick up object
- Crawls up a few steps
- Runs
- Makes marks with crayon
- Drops object into and takes it out of a cup

•••••••••• **At 18 Months (72 Weeks, or 1½ Years)** ••••••••••

Social
- Engages with others for play
- Helps dress and undress self
- Points to pictures in book or to object of interest to draw parent's attention to it
- Turns to look at adult if something new happens
- Begins to scoop with a spoon
- Uses words to ask for help

Language
- Identifies at least 2 body parts
- Names at least 5 familiar objects

Motor
- Walks up steps with 2 feet per step when hand is held
- Sits in a small chair
- Carries toy when walking
- Scribbles spontaneously
- Throws a small ball a few feet while standing

Social

▸ Plays alongside other children
▸ Takes off some clothing
▸ Scoops well with a spoon

Language

▸ Uses at least 50 words
▸ Combines 2 words into short phrase or sentence
▸ Follows 2-part instructions
▸ Names at least 5 body parts
▸ Speaks in words that are about 50% understandable by strangers

Motor

▸ Kicks a ball
▸ Jumps off the ground with 2 feet
▸ Runs with coordination
▸ Climbs up a ladder at a playground
▸ Stacks objects
▸ Turns book pages
▸ Uses hands to turn objects such as knobs, toys, or lids
▸ Draws lines

Social

▸ Urinates in a potty or toilet
▸ Spears food with fork
▸ Washes and dries hands
▸ Increasingly engages in imaginary play
▸ Tries to get parents to watch by saying, "Look at me!"

Language

▸ Uses pronouns correctly

Motor

- ► Walks up steps, alternating feet
- ► Runs well without falling
- ► Copies a vertical line
- ► Grasps crayon with thumb and fingers instead of fist
- ► Catches large balls

························ **At 3 Years** ························

Social

- ► Enters bathroom and urinates by herself
- ► Puts on coat, jacket, or shirt without help
- ► Eats without help
- ► Engages in imaginative play
- ► Plays well with others and shares

Language

- ► Uses 3-word sentences
- ► Speaks in words that are understandable to strangers 75% of the time
- ► Tells you a story from a book or TV
- ► Compares things using words such as *bigger* or *shorter*
- ► Understands prepositions such as *on* or *under*

Motor

- ► Pedals a tricycle
- ► Climbs on and off couch or chair
- ► Jumps forward
- ► Draws a single circle
- ► Draws a person with head and 1 other body part
- ► Cuts with child scissors

At 4 Years

Social

- Enters bathroom and has bowel movement by himself
- Brushes teeth
- Dresses and undresses without much help
- Engages in well-developed imaginative play

Language

- Answers questions such as "What do you do when you are cold?" or "What do you do when you are you sleepy?"
- Uses 4-word sentences
- Speaks in words that are 100% understandable to strangers
- Draws recognizable pictures
- Follows simple rules when playing a board or card game
- Tells parent a story from a book

Motor

- Hops on one foot
- Climbs stairs while alternating feet without help
- Draws a person with at least 3 body parts
- Draws a simple cross
- Unbuttons and buttons medium-sized buttons
- Grasps pencil with thumb and fingers instead of fist

At 5 and 6 Years

Social

- Follows simple directions
- Dresses with little assistance

Language

- Has good language skills
- Can count to 10
- Names 4 or more colors

Motor
▸ Balances on one foot
▸ Hops and skips
▸ Is able to tie a knot
▸ Draws a person with at least 6 body parts
▸ Prints some letters and numbers
▸ Can copy a square and a triangle

At School Age

Ongoing Issues Your Child May Face

As preterm babies get older, some of them may face ongoing physical problems (such as asthma or cerebral palsy). They may also face developmental challenges (such as difficulties paying attention or lack of motor control). This may be especially true for babies who were very small at birth.

Once your child reaches school age, it will be important for you to work closely with his teacher and other school staff to identify any areas of concern. They can also help you find the right resources for help. If the school does not have the resources your child needs, his teachers can help you find local groups or programs to help him do well in school. You are not alone! Your child's teachers and health care team are dedicated to helping you meet all his health and educational needs.

All children will babble before they say real words. All children will pull up to a stand before they walk. We are sure that children will develop in these patterns. However, children can reach these stages in different ways and at different times. This is especially true if they were born preterm. Take some time to think about your child's development and answer the following questions. Contact your child's doctor if you have any questions about your child's development.

Your Child's Development

- How does my child like to communicate?
  - How does he let me know what he is thinking and feeling?
- How does my child like to explore how to use his body?
  - Does he prefer using his fingers and hands (small muscles)?
  - Does he prefer using his arms and legs (large muscles)?
- How does my child respond to new situations?
  - Does he jump right in?
  - Does he prefer to hang back and look around before he feels safe?
- How does my child like to explore?
  - What kinds of objects and activities interest him?
  - What do those interests tell me about him?
- What are my child's strengths?
- In what ways does my child need more support?

Chapter
6
Common Conditions, Concerns, and Equipment in the NICU

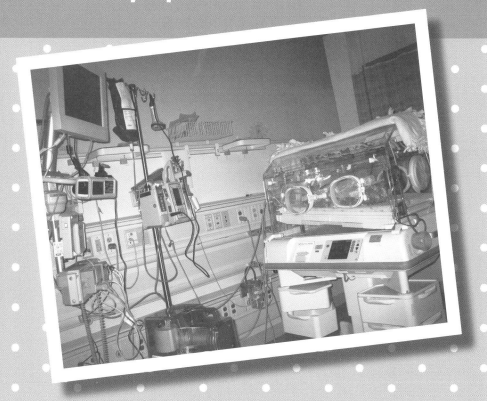

Babies in the NICU are carefully monitored because of the health risks they face. While this chapter lists common conditions babies in the NICU have or experience, it is by no means meant to scare parents. Not all preterm babies will have these problems, but, if your baby does have a common condition, the following explanation is meant to help you understand what is happening and calm your fears.

General Conditions

Prematurity

Babies born before 37 completed weeks of gestation (or before the 37th week of pregnancy) are called *preterm* (or *premature*). Preterm babies are at risk for a variety of problems, including

- Breathing concerns
- Feeding concerns (and breathing and feeding at the same time)
- Infection
- Staying warm

Preterm babies need special medical care that is offered only within NICUs or special care nurseries.

Heart and Blood Pressure Monitors

In the NICU, your baby's heart rate, respiratory (breathing) rate, blood pressure, and temperature will all be monitored. Small sticky pads are placed on your baby's skin, and these detect information and send it to a screen on a machine at your baby's bedside. A small blood pressure cuff is used to measure blood pressure. This is also hooked up to the machine. Sometimes, blood pressure is monitored through a thin tube inserted into an artery. An alarm will sound whenever your baby needs to be checked by a nurse, but some alarms are false alarms caused by your baby's movements.

Central Catheter (Line)

When your baby is born, the health care team may place a thin tube, called a central catheter or line, in the umbilical vein. This line is used to give your baby nutrition and medicine intravenously. The line also can be used to check how your baby is breathing. Later, your baby might need to have the umbilical line replaced with a peripherally inserted central catheter, or PICC, which is placed in one of the major blood vessels. Other types of central lines, such as Hickman and Broviac catheters, also may be needed.

Hyperbilirubinemia (Jaundice)

Hyperbilirubinemia, or jaundice, occurs when there is too much of a chemical called *bilirubin* in the blood. Bilirubin is made when red blood cells are broken down after normal use, as is common after a baby is born, or from an infection or problem with the blood. High levels of bilirubin cause the skin to become yellow or pink-yellow in color. The more bilirubin, the more yellow (or jaundiced) the skin becomes. If the bilirubin level becomes very, very high, it can cause more serious problems, like brain damage or hearing loss.

In a healthy baby, bilirubin moves through the blood to the liver and then leaves the body in the urine and stool. Because preterm babies have immature livers, there is a delay in how fast the bilirubin leaves the body. This can result in higher levels of bilirubin in a preterm baby than in a more mature baby. Bilirubin levels also can be higher in babies who are sick.

Bilirubin levels are measured in the blood shortly after birth and then every day until the levels begin to drop. Treatment for high bilirubin levels depends on your baby's weight and age. It usually includes using special blue lights, called phototherapy or "bili" lights. These lights change the bilirubin to make it more soluble so it can easily leave the body in the urine. During this treatment, your baby will lie under the lights. His eyes will be protected and his position will be changed frequently to expose all skin areas. How high the bilirubin levels are determines the number of lights a baby needs. If the phototherapy lights don't adequately decrease bilirubin levels, another treatment, called an *exchange transfusion,* can be done. This procedure is only rarely needed and involves exchanging some of the baby's blood with donated blood to lower the baby's bilirubin level.

Infection (Sepsis)

Sepsis is an infection of the bloodstream. Usually, it is caused by germs (bacteria). In some cases, it is caused by a virus or fungus.

Sepsis can be very serious and often requires additional care or longer hospital stays. When babies get ill in the first week after birth, the infection might have started before birth or during delivery. Babies who become ill after 7 days of age have what is known as *late-onset sepsis*. Preterm babies are at risk for infection because of their fragile skin and poor ability to fight off germs.

Possible Signs of Sepsis

- Body temperature that is too high or too low
- Breathing problems (such as apnea, or the need for oxygen or a ventilator)
- Change in blood pressure (especially low blood pressure)
- Low activity level or decreased movement
- Feeding problems

Treatment for Sepsis

- Antibiotics
- Blood tests to check for signs of infection
- Fluids or medicine to increase blood pressure
- Giving oxygen or using a ventilator to help the baby breathe

How long this treatment is needed depends on how sick the baby is and what caused the sepsis.

Temperature Control

Healthy, full-term babies have a layer of fat under the skin that protects them from heat loss. Babies who are born early have not had the chance to put on weight and do not have this fat layer under their skin. The best way to keep preterm babies warm is through the use of an incubator. This is a special crib that provides extra heat to preterm or sick babies. As your baby gets bigger and more mature, he will be able to move into an open crib. This is one of the main criteria used to determine when a baby is ready to go home.

Radiant Warmer

This is an open bed with a heat source over the baby. It may be used instead of an incubator, especially for babies who need frequent handling or care.

Late-Onset Hearing Loss: Extended Stay in NICU

Left undetected, hearing loss in babies can negatively affect speech and language acquisition, academic achievement, and social and emotional development. If detected early, however, morbidity can be diminished and even eliminated through Early Intervention services. This section reviews some of the risk factors associated with hearing loss that accompany a baby's extended stay in the NICU.

Very Low Birth Weight (<1,500 g)

The risk for sensorineural hearing loss increases as the birth weight decreases. Babies who weigh less than 1,500 g (3 lb 5 oz) at birth or are very sick at birth are at an increased risk for hearing loss.

Ototoxic Drugs

Ototoxic drugs can cause toxic reactions to structures of the inner ear, which can result in loss of hearing or balance. One example of an ototoxic drug is an aminoglycoside antibiotic. Aminoglycoside antibiotics may be ototoxic when administered to a child. They can also be ototoxic to a fetus when administered to a pregnant woman. Sensorineural hearing loss results from damage to the hair cells of the vestibular and cochlear organs (components of the inner ear).

Low Apgar Score (0–4 at 1 Minute or 1–6 at 5 Minutes)

Babies with low Apgar scores (see *Chapter 7, Glossary of NICU Terms*) are at a higher risk for hearing loss because of their existing condition or medical procedures that are needed to treat an existing condition.

Postnatal Infection Associated With Sensorineural Hearing Loss (Sepsis, Bacterial Meningitis)

Bacterial meningitis and sepsis are severe invasive diseases. These infections can lead to sensorineural hearing loss. In addition, antibiotics used to treat the infections may be ototoxic.

Hyperbilirubinemia Requiring Exchange Transfusion

Hyperbilirubinemia, or jaundice, occurs in 50% to 60% of all babies. It often causes no problems, but it can cause damage to the nervous system if it is severe. In cases of severe hyperbilirubinemia, the auditory neural pathways (cochlear nuclei of the brain stem) or the cochlea may be affected, leading to hearing loss. Babies with hyperbilirubinemia at a serum level requiring exchange transfusion should have additional auditory brain stem response, or ABR, testing.

Mechanical Ventilation for Longer Than 5 Days

By the time a baby has been put on mechanical ventilation, he may have already experienced a high level of oxygen deprivation. A lack of oxygen can accelerate the deterioration of the sensory cells of the inner ear. Mechanical ventilation also could indicate other possible problems associated with hearing loss, such as bronchopulmonary dysplasia (BPD) or persistent pulmonary hypertension of the newborn (PPHN; also known as persistent fetal circulation).

Condition at Birth Requiring Use of Extracorporeal Membrane Oxygenation

Babies who need extracorporeal membrane oxygenation (ECMO) may experience enough oxygen deprivation to cause damage to the sensory cells of the inner ear. About one-fourth of babies who receive ECMO develop sensorineural hearing loss. About half of babies who receive ECMO with sensorineural hearing loss have a progressive type of loss, which reinforces the importance of follow-up screening.

Permission to use information from Risk Factors for Late Onset Hearing Loss: Extended Stay in NICU *(**www.doh.wa.gov/Portals/1/Documents/Pubs/344-018_EHDDIRiskFactNICU-Detail.pdf**) was granted by the Washington State Department of Health Early Hearing Loss Detection, Diagnosis, and Intervention Program.*

Breathing Conditions

Apnea and Bradycardia

It is normal for preterm babies to have breathing pauses. Any pause in breathing that lasts for more than 20 seconds is called *apnea*. A decrease in a baby's heart rate below a normal level is called *bradycardia*. These conditions are common in preterm babies and usually go away when the babies reach between 35 and 40 weeks' adjusted age. However, apnea might take longer to go away in babies born very preterm (23–27 weeks' gestation). These conditions are common in preterm babies because the part of the brain that controls breathing is not fully developed. Apnea and bradycardia can cause the baby to become pale purple or dusky blue in color. The baby also might become limp, and his heart rate might slow down.

Babies in the NICU are watched closely for apnea and bradycardia (often called "As and Bs"). When a baby stops breathing or his heart rate drops below a certain number, a monitor alarm will sound.

There are several types of treatment. First, if the apnea and bradycardia are mild, the baby may simply need to be observed or gently reminded to breathe by touching him or changing his position. If the baby is very preterm or the apnea and bradycardia are severe, medicine (usually caffeine) is used. Otherwise, babies are treated with oxygen or air blowing in a little tube under their nose or with breathing support, such as CPAP or a ventilator.

Early Lung Conditions

Respiratory Distress Syndrome

Another term that you may hear is *respiratory distress syndrome* (RDS). It also might be called by its old name, hyaline membrane disease, or its biological cause, surfactant deficiency. Respiratory distress syndrome is very common in preterm babies. It affects babies whose lungs have lower than normal amounts of a body substance called *surfactant*. This substance helps make breathing easier by holding open the air sacs of the lungs. If these sacs do not open easily, the lungs cannot take in air, get oxygen into the bloodstream, or get rid of carbon dioxide. Babies with RDS breathe fast, causing the chest and ribs to pull in and out. They also may make grunting or soft crowing sounds when they breathe.

Tests to diagnose RDS include a chest radiograph and blood gas to measure oxygen and carbon dioxide levels in the blood. Any baby with trouble breathing should be checked for RDS.

Treatment includes giving the baby oxygen. This can be done with an oxygen hood or with CPAP. If oxygen isn't enough, a ventilator (breathing machine) is needed. To breathe on a ventilator, a tube must be placed into the baby's airway (trachea). This tube is needed to give surfactant and help with breathing. There are many different ventilators that may be used. Some give the baby regular breaths; others allow the baby to breathe on his own; and still others use gentle vibration to help the lungs. Up to 4 doses of surfactant can be given over the first 2 days after birth.

Complications of RDS can include lung collapse (pneumothorax), intraventricular hemorrhage (IVH), developmental delay, and BPD (also called chronic lung disease [CLD]).

Pneumothorax (Air Leaks or Lung Collapse)

A pneumothorax is an event that occurs when the breathing sacs in the lungs break and air leaks into and gets trapped in the space between the lung and the chest wall. If this happens, air cannot get back into the lungs for normal breathing. It can cause collapse of the lung as well. This condition is common in preterm babies or babies whose lungs lack surfactant. Babies who breathe in meconium (the first stool) while still in the womb are also at high risk for pneumothorax.

Three types of air leaks are seen in babies.

- *Spontaneous pneumothorax,* which occurs for no known reason in healthy babies and may or may not cause a problem.

- *Tension pneumothorax,* which is more common in babies who are on ventilators. This is a medical emergency because the lung collapse puts pressure on the heart, interfering with heart function and circulation.

- *Pulmonary interstitial emphysema,* which is a condition involving air leaking within the lung tissue itself. This type of air leak also puts the baby at increased risk of a pneumothorax and often requires the use of a special ventilator, especially a high-frequency ventilator.

Tests to diagnose a pneumothorax include the use of fiber-optic lights (transillumination) to look for trapped air in the lungs, chest radiographs, or both.

Treatment includes giving the baby high amounts of oxygen. A tension pneumothorax is treated with a chest tap (called a *thoracentesis*) to remove the air. If the air leak is severe, a chest tube is placed between the lung and chest wall to refill the lungs and allow them to heal over a few days.

Persistent Pulmonary Hypertension of the Newborn

Before birth, babies get oxygen from their mothers through the placenta. Therefore, they do not use their lungs to breathe air (although they make breathing movements, even when they are in the womb). When a baby is born, blood flows to the lungs and the baby breathes on his own. There are a number of conditions that can interrupt this process. Such interruptions are called PPHN. These include

- Infection
- Meconium aspiration (when a baby breathes in a small amount of stool while still in the womb)
- Low oxygen levels
- Lack of surfactant in the lungs

If blood does not go to the lungs, the baby does not have enough oxygen. This causes the baby's skin color to turn a bluish-gray color.

Tests to diagnose PPHN include checking the baby's blood oxygen, pH, and carbon dioxide levels (blood gases); chest radiographs; and a special study of baby's heart called an echocardiogram (sometimes referred to as an "echo"). This test checks the structure of the heart and lungs, as well as blood pressure.

Treatments include using a ventilator to help the baby breathe, blood pressure medicine, a medicine that relaxes the lung blood pressure (called nitric oxide), and, in some cases, heart-lung bypass (ECMO).

Transient Tachypnea of the Newborn

Tachypnea is the medical word for fast or rapid breathing. Rapid breathing that gets better over the first few hours or days and does not recur is called *transient tachypnea of the newborn* (TTN). This occurs because fluid in the baby's lungs is not absorbed after birth. The symptoms of TTN are similar to RDS but usually milder. Some babies with TTN need oxygen, but only rarely will a baby with TTN need to be on a ventilator.

Oxygen Hood and Nasal Cannula

An oxygen hood is a clear plastic box that goes over a baby's head. A nasal cannula is a thin tube with 2 small prongs that fit into a baby's nostrils. Both give oxygen to help with breathing.

Pulse Oximeter

To measure a baby's pulse, a small, stretchy bandage (oximeter) with a sensor in it is wrapped around the baby's foot, hand, or wrist. The oximeter uses a light sensor to make sure there is enough oxygen in the baby's blood. The sensor does not hurt the baby; it helps the health care team know if the baby needs more or less oxygen.

Later Lung Conditions

Bronchopulmonary Dysplasia

This also is known as CLD of prematurity. Bronchopulmonary dysplasia is most common in babies who

- Lack surfactant in their lungs.
- Have very underdeveloped lungs.
- Need high amounts of oxygen.
- Are on a ventilator.

The highest rates of BPD are among babies born at 23 to 26 weeks of gestation (14–17 weeks before their due date). However, it can occur in other preterm babies as well. Rarely, BPD can affect full-term babies who are ill.

Treatment includes giving the baby oxygen, good nutrition, and, sometimes, diuretics (medicine that increases urine output) or bronchodilators (medicine that helps open the airways). A baby with BPD might need to be on a ventilator for a while before he can breathe on his own. After the ventilator is removed, the baby still will need to get oxygen through a little tube under the nose. Some babies need to go home with this extra oxygen.

A baby with BPD must be protected from catching a cold or the flu. For these babies, a simple cold can turn into a severe, or even fatal, pneumonia. While many babies with BPD outgrow their lung problems, some preterm babies with BPD will have lung problems that last through young adulthood.

Pneumonia
Pneumonia is a common lung infection in preterm and other sick babies. A baby's doctors may suspect pneumonia if the baby has difficulty breathing, if his rate of breathing changes, or if he has an increased number of apnea episodes.

The doctor will listen to the baby's lungs with a stethoscope and then obtain a radiograph to see if there is excess fluid in the lungs. Sometimes, the doctor may insert a thin tube down the windpipe (trachea) to take a sample of the lung fluid. The fluid is then tested to see what type of bacterium or virus is causing the infection, so that the doctor can choose the most effective drug to treat it. Babies with pneumonia generally are treated with antibiotics. They also may need additional oxygen until the infection clears up.

Heart Conditions

Patent Ductus Arteriosus
Before birth, babies get oxygen from their mothers. They do not use their lungs to breathe. Instead, blood goes past the lungs through an opening in a blood vessel just outside the heart called the *ductus arteriosus.* During the first few hours or days after birth, this opening starts to close, allowing the baby to use his lungs to breathe. However, it is not uncommon for the ductus arteriosus to stay open in sick or preterm babies. If that happens, it is called a patent ductus arteriosus (PDA). (The ductus is actually a normal fetal artery connecting the aorta and the pulmonary artery.)

In a PDA, extra fluid builds up in the lungs, making it hard for the baby to breathe. Symptoms include

- Fast breathing
- Need of a ventilator (breathing machine)
- Poor growth
- Presence of a heart murmur

Treatment depends on how the baby is affected by the PDA. A cardiologist (heart doctor) will examine the baby and use a heart test called an echocardiogram to confirm the PDA. A medicine may be used to close the PDA. In some cases, the baby might need to have surgery to close the PDA.

Congenital Heart Defects

Congenital heart defects are structural heart problems that are present at birth. They originate in the first weeks of pregnancy when the heart is forming.

Coarctation of the Aorta

The aorta is the large artery that sends blood from the heart to the rest of the body. In this condition, the aorta may be too narrow for the blood to flow evenly. A surgeon can remove the narrow part and connect the ends together, replace the constricted section with artificial material, or patch it with part of a blood vessel taken from elsewhere in the body. Sometimes, this narrowed area can be widened by inflating a balloon on the tip of a catheter inserted through an artery.

Heart Valve Abnormalities

Some babies are born with heart valves that are narrowed, closed, or blocked and prevent blood from flowing smoothly. Some babies may require placement of a shunt (tube between 2 blood vessels) to allow blood to bypass the blockage until the baby is big enough to have the valve repaired or replaced.

Septal Defect

A septal defect refers to a hole in the wall (septum) that divides the 2 upper or lower chambers of the heart. Because of this hole, the blood cannot circulate as it should, and the heart has to work extra hard. A surgeon can close the hole by sewing or patching it. Small holes might close by themselves and not need repair at all.

Tetralogy of Fallot

In tetralogy of Fallot, a combination of 4 structural problems keeps the normal amount of blood from getting to the lungs. As a result, the baby has episodes of cyanosis (blue spells) and may grow poorly. New surgical techniques allow early repair of this complex heart defect.

Transposition of the Great Arteries

With transposition of the great arteries, the positions of the 2 major arteries leaving the heart are reversed. Each artery arises from the wrong pumping chamber. Surgical advances have enabled correction of this problem in the first month after birth.

Intestinal Conditions

Necrotizing Enterocolitis

Necrotizing enterocolitis (NEC) is a serious disease of the intestines that most often affects preterm babies; however, sometimes, full-term babies also get NEC. Babies who are born very early, are very small, or are very sick are at highest risk. This is because they often have less blood flow to their intestines and are at higher risk for infection.

Necrotizing enterocolitis usually develops within the first 3 weeks after birth, often after feedings are started. The intestine becomes smaller and weaker, and this can cause a hole (perforation) to form. If a hole develops, bacteria can leak into the baby's blood or abdomen, causing a life-threatening infection.

Necrotizing enterocolitis can happen very quickly—within a few hours. A baby can rapidly go from healthy to critically ill. When a baby recovers from NEC, the bowel may still be weak, and additional problems can come up when feedings are started again.

Tests for NEC include abdominal radiographs and blood tests.

Treatment includes giving the baby IV fluids and antibiotics. Babies with NEC may have a tube inserted by surgeons to drain stomach acid and are fed through an IV to let the bowels rest (often for 1–2 weeks). Surgery is needed if the disease is severe or a hole is found in the intestine.

Blood Conditions

Anemia

Anemia is the term for a low blood cell count or low level of red blood cells. Red blood cells are important because they carry oxygen throughout the body. Preterm babies are at higher risk for anemia because their red blood cells have shortened survival compared with full-term babies and because of the number of blood tests they need. If anemia is severe or the baby also has low blood pressure, a blood transfusion might be needed. Less severe anemia is treated by giving iron medicine and by adding iron to breast milk or formula.

Neurological Conditions

Intraventricular Hemorrhage

An IVH is a collection of blood (hemorrhage) in or around the normally fluid-filled spaces (ventricles) on each side of the brain. It is common in very small and very sick preterm babies because the blood vessels on their brains are very delicate and can break easily. Babies with breathing problems and low blood pressure are at especially high risk for IVH. Most hemorrhages occur in the first few days after birth. Babies born before 32 weeks' gestation have a special test of the head (sonogram or ultrasound) by the seventh day of age. Intraventricular hemorrhage is divided into 4 grades (or degrees).

- **Grade 1:** a small amount of blood outside the ventricles
- **Grade 2:** bleeding inside the ventricles, but the ventricles are normal size
- **Grade 3:** blood inside the ventricles, and the ventricles are large in size
- **Grade 4:** bleeding outside the ventricles into the surrounding brain tissue

Major bleeding can cause increased pressure on the brain. It also can cause not enough blood to go to the brain tissue. Brain bleeding in preterm babies can have a variety of long-term effects. Some babies will not have any permanent damage and will develop normally. Other babies can have mild, moderate, or severe brain damage. Depending on severity, IVH might need further neurosurgical treatment, like ventriculoperitoneal (or VP) shunts.

Brain and Body Imaging

There are several types of tests that your baby may need to help doctors see inside his body, including

- **Ultrasound:** Takes pictures of the internal organs using sound waves. It does not hurt and can be done at the baby's bedside.

- **Radiographs (also called x-rays):** Takes pictures of the lungs, bones, and other internal organs. Several radiographs might be needed depending on what the doctor is looking for. The baby will be exposed to a small amount of radiation (x-rays) during a radiograph. However, radiographs are often needed to help make important decisions about a baby's care. They also can be done at the bedside.

- **Computed tomography (CT; also sometimes called a CAT scan):** Takes more detailed pictures than a radiograph or an ultrasound. A beam of energy is focused on a certain area of the body and then shown in detail on a computer. This test cannot be done at the baby's bedside and involves greater radiation exposure than a regular radiograph.

- **Magnetic resonance imaging (MRI):** Uses powerful magnets and computers to create images of tissue that are even more detailed than CT. This test cannot be done at the baby's bedside. Some babies need sedation to help keep them still during this test. An MRI does not expose the baby to any radiation.

Periventricular Leukomalacia

Periventricular leukomalacia (PVL) is a cyst formation in the brain tissue around the ventricles (chambers) in the brain. It may be caused by

- A hemorrhage in the brain
- A brain infection, such as meningitis
- Other infections, including infections during the prenatal period

It can occur in preterm babies and usually happens without warning. It can be seen with a head ultrasound, although it may take several weeks before PVL shows up. Periventricular leukomalacia increases the risk of a baby having long-term problems with muscle movement and coordination, vision, or intellectual development.

Retinopathy of Prematurity

Retinopathy of prematurity (ROP) is an abnormal growth of blood vessels in the retina (the lining at the back of the eyeball that sends images to the brain). It is seen in some preterm babies, especially those born more than 12 weeks early.

When a baby is born early, the blood vessels in the eyes are not fully developed. If these blood vessels do not grow normally, bleeding and scarring can affect vision. Doctors do not know all the reasons why ROP happens, but being preterm and the use of high amounts of oxygen are 2 risk factors. This is why oxygen levels for preterm babies are tightly controlled.

Retinopathy of prematurity is more common in very small and very preterm babies. If your baby was born before 30 weeks' gestation, he will need to see a specially trained eye doctor called an ophthalmologist. The doctor will look at the development of your baby's retina (eye). Regular eye examinations will be needed until the retina is fully developed. Severe ROP can lead to vision problems and even blindness. Treatment may involve laser surgery or cryosurgery to stop the blood vessels from growing abnormally.

Chapter
7
Glossary of NICU Terms

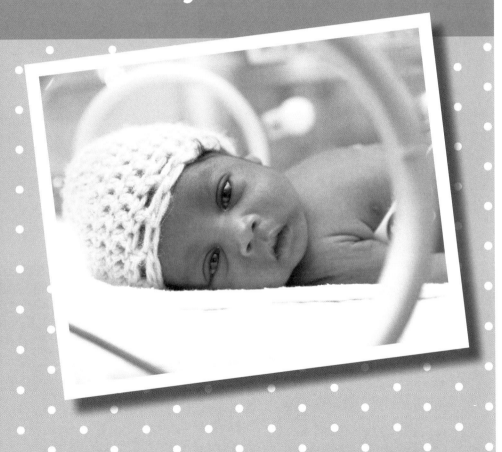

Glossary definitions are adapted from the March of Dimes and Raising Multiples (formerly known as Mothers of Supertwins [MOST]).

ABO incompatibility
Blood incompatibility between the mother and fetus that can result in destruction of fetal red blood cells, jaundice, and anemia.

Adjusted age
Used most appropriately to describe newborns, infants, and children as old as 3 years who were born preterm. Also called "corrected age," adjusted age is calculated by subtracting the number of weeks born before 40 weeks of gestation from the chronological age.

Anemia
One of the more common blood disorders, anemia occurs when the level of healthy red blood cells in the body becomes too low.

Apgar score
A scoring system that helps the physician estimate a baby's general condition at birth. The test measures a baby's heart rate, breathing, muscle tone, reflex response, and color at 1 minute, 5 minutes, and 10 minutes after birth. Named after its creator, Virginia Apgar.

Apnea
A pause in breathing that lasts longer than 20 seconds. Apnea of prematurity occurs in babies who are born preterm (<34 weeks of gestation). Because the brain or respiratory system may be immature or underdeveloped, the baby may not be able to regulate his or her own breathing.

Apnea monitor
Machine that detects interruptions in breathing.

Artery
Blood vessel that carries blood away from the heart to all parts of the body.

Asphyxia
Lack of oxygen.

Aspiration
Inhaling a foreign object, such as food, medicine, or meconium.

Attending physician
The physician who has been selected by or assigned to the patient and who has assumed primary responsibility for the treatment and care of the patient.

Audiologist
A medical professional with 6 years of training who treats patients with hearing, balance, and related ear problems.

Bagging
Pumping air or oxygen into a baby's lungs by squeezing a bag or air into a mask placed over the baby's mouth and nose or through an endotracheal tube.

Betamethasone

Corticosteroid given to the mother before the baby is born to stimulate fetal lung maturation and to decrease the frequency and damage from intracranial hemorrhage in preterm babies.

"Bili" lights

Blue fluorescent lights used to treat jaundice.

Bilirubin

A breakdown product of hemoglobin, the substance in blood that carries oxygen. Normally, bilirubin passes through the liver and is excreted as bile through the intestine. Jaundice occurs when bilirubin builds up faster than a newborn's liver can break it down and pass it from the body.

Birth defect

Abnormality of structure, function, or body metabolism (inborn error of body chemistry) present at birth that results in physical or mental disability or is fatal.

Blood gases

Levels of oxygen and carbon dioxide in the blood.

Bradycardia

A heart rate of less than 100 beats per minute, slower than normal for a baby.

Breast pump

A machine to collect human (breast) milk without the baby present. A hospital-grade breast pump is often more powerful than those for home use and may be available for rental.

Bronchopulmonary dysplasia (BPD)

A chronic lung disorder that is most common among children who were born preterm, with low birth weights, and who received prolonged mechanical ventilation.

Cannula

A slender tube that sits below the nose and can be used to deliver oxygen.

Cardiopulmonary monitor

Machine that tracks heart and breathing rates.

Catheter

A hollow, flexible tube for insertion into a body cavity, duct, or vessel to allow the passage of fluids, or distend or drain a passageway or body cavity. Its uses include delivery of intravenous fluids, drainage of urine from the bladder through the urethra, or insertion through a blood vessel into the heart for diagnostic purposes.

Central venous line

A narrow tube that is placed into a blood vessel and passed into a larger blood vessel in the chest or abdomen. It is used to deliver medicine and intravenous nutrition and to draw blood.

Cerebral palsy

Appearing in the first few years after birth, this diagnosis means the child will have abnormal muscle tone (too tight or too loose) and might also have problems moving parts of his body. The extent of the problem may not be fully known until about age 2 years.

Complete blood cell count (CBC)
Blood test that looks at the number and type of white blood cells (infection-fighting cells), the concentration of hemoglobin, the percentage of blood volume consisting of red blood cells (hematocrit, oxygen-carrying cells), and the number of platelets (blood-clotting cells).

Computed tomography (CT)
Imaging technique that produces precise pictures of tissue using a narrow beam of radiation and computer processing of a series of images. Also sometimes called a CAT scan.

Congenital diaphragmatic hernia
Birth defect involving an opening in the diaphragm, the large muscle that separates the chest and abdomen. Abdominal organs, such as the stomach, liver, and intestines, can move through the opening into the chest, where they interfere with lung development.

Continuous positive airway pressure (CPAP)
This machine pushes a continuous flow of air or oxygen, through small tubes that fit into a baby's nostrils (called nasal CPAP) or through a tube that has been inserted into the windpipe, to the airways to help keep tiny air passages in the lungs open. The tubes are attached to a ventilator, which helps the baby breathe but does not breathe for him.

Cryotherapy
Freezing of abnormal tissue to halt its growth. This form of treatment can be used in severe cases of retinopathy of prematurity (ROP), but, more recently, cryotherapy for ROP has been largely replaced by laser therapy.

Cubic centimeter (cm³)
A metric unit of volume equal to a milliliter (mL). There are 30 cm^3 in a fluid ounce.

Culture
A laboratory test that detects infections in the body by placing samples in special nutrients that allow bacteria to grow. Most current culture systems monitor bacterial growth for up to 7 days.

Cyanosis
A blue or gray discoloration of the skin caused by insufficient oxygen.

Cytomegalovirus (CMV)
A viral infection that, when contracted by a pregnant woman, can result in severe newborn illness and sometimes lead to chronic disabilities, such as intellectual disability, or vision and hearing loss. Also can be acquired after birth and can lead to hearing loss.

Developmental delay
The failure to meet certain milestones, such as rolling, sitting, walking, and talking, at the typical age.

Developmental pediatrician
These physicians have 10 years of training and specialize in evaluating and treating problems with child development. They assess the level of development of preterm babies from the motor (movement) and intellectual (learning) viewpoints.

Early Intervention program
Refers to services that are provided to children aged 3 years or younger who have or might develop a special need that may affect their development.

Echocardiogram
The use of ultrasound to view the structure and function of the heart. Sometimes referred to as "echo."

Electrocardiogram (ECG)
Measurement of electrical activity of the heart from a number of specific viewpoints. This activity is detected through adhesive patches placed on the chest, arms, and legs.

Electrodes
A conductor used to make contact with a nonmetallic part of a circuit.

Electroencephalogram (EEG)
A noninvasive and painless study in which electrodes placed on the scalp record the electrical activity of the brain. To conduct the study, metal electrodes have to be temporarily glued to the scalp.

Endotracheal tube
A tube that is placed down a newborn's trachea (windpipe) and delivers warm humidified air and oxygen to the lungs.

Exchange transfusion
Special type of blood transfusion in which some of the baby's blood is removed and replaced with blood from a donor. It can be used to treat severe jaundice.

Extracorporeal membrane oxygenation (ECMO)
In babies, this machine usually is used to allow the lungs to rest and recover from disease or medical conditions. Similar to a heart-lung bypass performed in the operating room for heart surgery but, in newborns, it is used for longer periods. Also called extracorporeal life support (ECLS).

Extremely low birth weight
Babies with a birth weight of less than 1,000 g (2 lb 3 oz).

Extremely preterm
Babies born between 23 and 27 weeks' gestation.

Failure to thrive
The failure to gain weight as expected, which is often accompanied by poor height growth.

Fellow

Physician who has completed medical school, internship, and a residency and currently is undergoing very specialized (subspecialty) training in one particular field of study. For example, neonatology fellows are training to become sub-specialists in neonatal medicine.

Fontanelle

Soft spot between the parts of a baby's skull that will later grow together. Also spelled fontanel.

Gastroenterologist

A physician with specialized training in diagnosing and treating diseases of the gastrointestinal tract and digestive system.

Gastroesophageal reflux

Occurs when gastric juice from the stomach backs up into the esophagus. Adults refer to this as "heartburn," although it has nothing to do with the heart.

Gastrointestinal tract

The tube that goes from the mouth to the anus, where food is digested and eliminated from the body (as a bowel movement). Also called GI tract.

Gastroschisis

Birth defect involving an opening in the abdominal wall, through which the abdominal organs bulge out, usually right beside the umbilical cord.

Gastrostomy

Surgically created opening through the abdominal skin and into the stomach, through which a baby can be fed.

Gavage

A method of feeding a baby with human (breast) milk or formula before he has learned how to coordinate breathing and swallowing. A small, flexible tube is placed into a baby's nostril or mouth and passed down into the stomach.

Gestation

Period between the mother's last menstrual period and the baby's birth. In humans, 40 weeks is the average gestation for a full-term singleton. Commonly called pregnancy.

Gram (g)

A metric unit of weight equal to one-thousandth of a kilogram. One gram weighs the same as one plain candy-coated chocolate piece or one small paper clip. There are approximately 30 g in 1 oz.

Group B streptococcus

Bacterial infection that a baby can contract as he passes through the birth canal, which sometimes results in further illness. Many cases can be prevented by screening and treating infected women with antibiotics during labor and delivery.

Heart failure
When the heart cannot pump enough blood to meet the body's needs.

Hematocrit
The percentage of blood volume consisting of red blood cells. Used as a measure of anemia.

Hemoglobin
The component of red blood cells that carries oxygen. Used as a measure of anemia.

Hernia
The protrusion of an organ or structure through muscles that usually contain them.

Herpes simplex
Viral infection that can be transmitted sexually, sometimes causing genital sores in infected adults. The virus (human herpesvirus 1 or 2) can occupy the mouth, genitals, or birth canal; on the lips it causes cold sores. A baby may become infected passing through an infected birth canal, which sometimes results in severe newborn illness or future medical problems.

High-frequency ventilation
Special form of mechanical ventilation that is designed to help reduce complications to a baby's delicate lungs. It provides rapid respiratory rates. Often called an oscillator or a jet ventilator (respirator).

Hydrocephalus
A condition in which too much fluid collects in the ventricles, exerting increased pressure on the brain and causing a baby's head to expand abnormally. Surgery may be required.

Hyperglycemia
High blood glucose levels.

Hypoglycemia
Low blood glucose levels.

Ileal perforation
A hole in part of the small intestine called the ileum.

Incubator
A heat-controlled crib used to maintain a baby's body temperature in the normal range. Also known as an Isolette (a trademarked term).

Inflammation
Pain, redness, and swelling, possibly caused by infection or injury.

Infusion pump
Device that delivers measured amounts of fluids or medicines into the bloodstream over a period of time.

Interval delivery
In multiple gestation, the delivery of a subsequent baby that is delayed after the preterm delivery of the first baby.

Intrauterine growth restriction (IUGR)
Inadequate growth of the fetus so that it is smaller than expected for gestational age. This can happen at any time during pregnancy.

Intravenous (IV)
A small tube inserted into a vein in the hand, foot, arm, leg, or scalp. An IV delivers medicine and/or fluids into the blood.

Intraventricular hemorrhage (IVH)
Condition in which immature and fragile blood vessels within the brain bleed into the hollow chambers (ventricles) normally reserved for cerebrospinal fluid. Sometimes this bleeding also spreads into the tissue surrounding the ventricles. An IVH is assigned a grade (1–4) to give an estimate of how serious it is.

Intubation
The procedure of inserting a tube through the mouth or nose, down the throat, and into the trachea or windpipe of a patient who may have difficulty breathing or might be at risk of stopping breathing because of illness, surgery, or other medical problem.

Jaundice
Yellow discoloration of skin and, sometimes, whites of the eyes that results from an excess of a body chemical called bilirubin in the body's system. If it is significant, jaundice might require use of special lights (phototherapy) until the baby is more mature. Severe jaundice is treated with exchange transfusion. Also known as hyperbilirubinemia.

Kangaroo care
See Skin-to-skin (kangaroo) care.

Lactation consultant
A health care professional (sometimes, but not always, a nurse) who provides information and support about breast-feeding and pumping breast milk.

Lanugo
Fine, downy hair that covers the fetus until shortly before or after birth.

Late-preterm baby
A baby born 4 to 6 weeks before his due date.

Lead wires
The wires that go from a monitor to its electrodes (sticky patches on the chest).

Lesion
A patch of abnormal skin, or the part of an injury or infection that is abnormal and causes an illness.

Licensed practical nurse (LPN)
Health care professional with a vocational education lasting approximately 12 months and licensed to give nursing care under the direct supervision of a registered nurse or physician. In some states, called a licensed vocational nurse (LVN).

Ligation
The act of binding or of applying a tie, wire, or bandage around a limb or blood vessel to restrict blood flow. It is used to treat patent ductus arteriosus, among other uses.

Liquid ventilation
A form of respiration in which a machine is used to deliver an oxygen-rich liquid, rather than air.

Low birth weight
Babies who are born weighing less than 2,500 g (5 lb 8 oz).

Lumbar puncture
A diagnostic procedure that is done to collect a sample of spinal fluid for analysis or, on rare occasions, to relieve increased pressure in the spinal fluid. It is also known as a spinal tap.

Magnetic resonance imaging (MRI)
Imaging technique that uses powerful magnets and computers to produce a detailed picture of internal tissues and organs.

Mechanical ventilation
Using a ventilator to help a very sick baby breathe while his lungs recover.

Meconium
Fecal material made by the fetus; usually passed in the first bowel movement after birth. Sometimes meconium is passed in the amniotic fluid before birth and inhaled in the amniotic fluid during the fetus's normal breathing movement.

Meconium aspiration syndrome
Problems caused by meconium (baby's first bowel movement) going into the lungs while the baby is still in the womb. This can be serious, but the baby usually eventually recovers fully.

Medicaid
A program partially sponsored by the federal government and administered by states that is intended to provide health care and health-related services to low-income individuals and other qualifying persons. A child may qualify regardless of parental income, based on medical circumstances, even if the child has other health insurance.

Meningitis
An inflammation of the lining of the brain, usually from viral or bacterial infection.

Microcephaly
A condition in which the circumference of the head is small because of abnormal brain growth. This condition might result in future cerebral palsy or learning problems.

Micro-preemie
Baby who is born weighing less than 800 g (1 lb 12 oz).

Milestones
Skills most children can perform at certain ages. Examples include smiling, rolling, sitting, scooting, crawling, standing, walking, and talking.

Monitor

A machine that records information such as heartbeat, body temperature, respiration rate, and blood pressure.

Moro reflex

A normal reflex of young babies; a sudden loud noise causes the baby to stretch out the arms and flex (scrunch up) the legs.

Myopia

The inability to see distant objects as clearly as near objects.

Nasal cannula

The "oxygen tubes" that give extra oxygen by blowing moisturized oxygen, possibly mixed with air, into the nose.

Nasal prongs

Small plastic tubes that fit into or under a baby's nose to deliver oxygen.

Nasogastric tube

A tube that is passed through the nose and down through the throat and esophagus and into the stomach.

Nebulizer treatment

A device for giving medicine by making a fine mist that is inhaled through the nose and/or mouth.

Necrotizing enterocolitis (NEC)

An infection that destroys part of the baby's intestines. Drugs and/or surgery may be required.

Neonatal intensive care unit (NICU)

There are 4 levels of NICU. Level 1 is a well-baby nursery and requires pediatricians, family physicians, nurse practitioners, and other advanced practice registered nurses. Level 2 is a special care nursery and requires pediatric hospitalists, a neonatologist, and neonatal nurse practitioners in addition to level 1 providers. Level 3 is a NICU that requires pediatric medical subspecialists, pediatric anesthesiologists, pediatric surgeons, and pediatric ophthalmologists. Level 4, a regional perinatal center, requires pediatric surgical subspecialists in addition to the providers required in level 3.

Neonatal nurse practitioner (NNP)

An advanced practice nurse with specialized training and expertise in neonatal care, NNPs are licensed to assess, diagnose, manage, and treat critically ill and convalescing neonates. In addition, NNPs prescribe medicine, write orders, interpret results, perform emergency and daily procedures, and attend high-risk deliveries.

Neonatologist

Physician with at least 6 additional years of post–medical school training specialized in dealing with the diseases and care of newborns.

Neurologist

Physician with at least 3 years of post–medical school training specialized in dealing with the diseases and care of the brain and nerves.

Nitric oxide
A gas naturally produced by the body that can also be given as a medicine that is breathed in and helps expand blood vessels. It is sometimes used to treat babies with persistent pulmonary hypertension of the newborn.

Noninvasive
Something that does not enter the body through the skin or an opening such as the mouth, nose, or anus.

Occupational therapist (OT)
A health care professional with 4 to 6 years of training who helps people who are ill or disabled learn to manage their daily activities. In the neonatal intensive care unit, OTs may be involved in giving the preterm baby stimulation and helping the baby learn to coordinate sucking, breathing, and swallowing while helping the baby stay comfortable and relaxed. Also teach parents about techniques to enhance baby development and other activities.

Ophthalmologist
Physician (MD) specializing in diagnosis and treatment of eye diseases and disorders refractive, medical, and surgical problems.

Orogastric tube
A flexible tube inserted through the mouth, down the throat and esophagus, and into the stomach.

Otoacoustic emission test
A passive audiologic test that verifies cochlear activity; often used in testing babies suspected of hearing loss.

Oxygen hood and nasal cannula
An oxygen hood is a clear plastic box that goes over a baby's head. A nasal cannula is a thin tube with 2 small prongs that fit into a baby's nostrils. Both give oxygen to help with breathing.

Oxygen therapy
Giving extra oxygen to the tissues of the body through the lungs in a number of ways, including through a ventilator (respirator), mask, nasal cannula, or plastic oxygen hood or tent. The amount of oxygen given may be measured as a percentage and in number of liters, or milliliters, of flow per minute.

Patent ductus arteriosus (PDA)
A heart condition caused by the failure of a small blood vessel (the ductus arteriosus) to close. Usually, this normal opening between the aorta and pulmonary artery closes just after birth. When it does not, the baby may be treated with medicine or surgery to fix the condition, which prevents too much blood from "flooding" the lungs.

Pediatrician
Physician with at least 3 post–medical school years of training in the care and treatment of newborns, infants, children, and adolescents.

Peripherally inserted central catheter (PICC)

A long catheter placed into a surface vein, with the catheter tip extending farther into the body into a large central vein. A PICC does not have to be replaced as often as a regular intravenous catheter (line).

Periventricular leukomalacia

Changes, usually small cysts, in brain tissue around the ventricles or fluid spaces of the brain. This cystic change is linked with an increased risk of future problems with learning, vision, or movement.

Persistent pulmonary hypertension

of the newborn (PPHN)

With PPHN, it is difficult for blood to get into the lungs and pick up more oxygen that can go to the rest of the body. The cause is usually unknown, and treatments are based on the individual situation. Also known as persistent fetal circulation.

Phototherapy

Treatment for jaundice in a newborn. The newborn is placed under (or on top of) special lights to help the body break down the extra bilirubin in the blood.

Physical therapist (PT)

A health care professional with 4 years or more of training who performs and teaches exercises and other physical activities to aid in rehabilitation and maximize physical muscle and movement development.

Physician

A graduate of allopathic medical school or school of osteopathy with an MD or DO degree.

Pneumothorax

Air that has leaked from a baby's lungs and gets trapped in the space between the baby's lungs and chest wall. While small leaks usually cause no problems and require no treatment, larger leaks may cause serious complications, such as lung collapse, and require withdrawal of the air with a needle and syringe or a surgical procedure to place a tube to drain the trapped air and reinflate the lung.

Preemie

A commonly heard term for a baby born preterm.

Preterm

Baby born before 37 completed weeks of gestation. Also called premature.

Pulse oximeter

A small device worn on the finger, toe, or earlobe that uses a light sensor to painlessly help determine levels of oxygen in the blood.

Radiant warmer

A heater that works by sending out radiant energy, usually in the form of heat. It warms objects without needing to touch them. Radiant warmers are often used to maintain temperature of babies in the neonatal intensive care unit.

Radiologist
A physician with 7 years of training who specializes in creating and interpreting pictures of areas inside the body.

Registered nurse (RN)
Health care professional with 2 or 4 years of training who is licensed to treat patient responses to illness and to carry out medicine regimens prescribed by a physician, nurse practitioner, dentist, or physician assistant. Usually has an associate's or bachelor's degree and may have additional degrees or certificates when working in the neonatal intensive care unit.

Resident
A physician who is in the process of completing the additional 3 years of training in a specialty (for example, pediatrics, ophthalmology, radiology, obstetrics/gynecology) following medical school.

Respirator
A machine that helps breathing by supplying and regulating a flow of air and oxygen that goes through a tube threaded through the nose or mouth, down the back of the throat, and into the trachea (windpipe). It is also called a ventilator.

Respiratory distress syndrome (RDS)
Condition in which a preterm baby with immature lungs does not have sufficient surfactant, a protective film that helps air sacs in the lungs to stay open.

Respiratory syncytial virus (RSV)
A virus that causes a mild, cold-like illness in adults. In preterm or full-term babies with lung problems, it can cause serious illness, such as bronchiolitis or pneumonia.

Respiratory therapist
A health care professional with 3 to 5 years of training who assesses breathing and heart function, treats with oxygen therapy or ventilation, and gives medicines to help with breathing as prescribed by a physician or practitioner.

Retina
Lining at the rear of the eye that relays messages about what the eyes see to the brain.

Retinopathy of prematurity (ROP)
A condition in which the blood vessels in a baby's eyes do not develop normally. This can reverse and normalize or progress to serious disease that can lead to hemorrhage, scarring, or retinal detachment that limits vision. Treated with laser therapy.

Rh disease
Blood incompatibility between the mother and fetus that causes destruction of fetal red blood cells.

Sepsis
A blood infection.

Skin-to-skin (kangaroo) care
Holding a baby against one's naked chest, so there is skin-to-skin contact.

Small for gestational age (SGA)
Babies whose birth weight is less than the 10th percentile for their gestational age. If weight gain of the fetus is abnormal, this is called intrauterine growth restriction.

Social worker
A professional with 4 to 6 years of training who helps families cope with stress, crisis, and change. In the neonatal intensive care unit setting, the social worker helps families access community resources, such as support groups and assistance programs. Social workers also help with planning the baby's hospital discharge.

Spina bifida
A birth defect involving the spinal cord, often resulting in varying degrees of paralysis and bladder and bowel problems. Affected babies may require surgery during the newborn period to close the back and prevent further nerve damage and infection. Surgery cannot reverse nerve damage that already has occurred.

Step-down unit
Nursing unit with patients who are not in need of intensive care but still require skilled nursing care.

Supplemental Security Income (SSI)
A federal income program funded by general tax revenues. Parents of children who qualify, based on medical and financial criteria, receive monthly payments to assist with health care expenses.

Surfactant/pulmonary surfactant
A protective substance that keeps small air sacs in the lungs from collapsing.

Swaddling
Wrapping babies snugly in cloths or blankets so that movement of the limbs is restricted, providing the baby with a secure, womb-like feeling.

Syndrome
A combination of signs and symptoms that, when present together, are associated with a specific medical condition.

Tachycardia
Rapid heart rate.

Tachypnea
Rapid breathing.

Tonic neck reflex
One of the reflexes present at birth. A baby will bend one arm while the other is extended away from the body, in the direction the baby is facing. Also called the fencing reflex.

Total parenteral nutrition (TPN)
A technique in which nutrients are given to a person through an intravenous infusion.Often requires a peripherally inserted central catheter.

Toxoplasmosis
A parasitic infection that, when contracted by a pregnant woman, can result in serious newborn illness and chronic disabilities, such as intellectual disability, cerebral palsy, seizures, or vision and hearing loss.

Transfusion
The transfer of whole blood or blood products from one individual to another.

Twin-twin transfusion syndrome
A disease of the placenta (or afterbirth) that affects identical twin pregnancies. The shared placenta contains abnormal blood vessels that can convey blood from one twin to another, resulting in a higher red blood cell count and, sometimes, better growth in one twin than another.

Ultrasound (sonogram)
The use of ultrasonic waves for diagnostic or therapeutic purposes. In the neonatal intensive care unit, ultrasound is used to obtain an image of an internal body structure.

Umbilical arterial catheter (UAC)
A line placed directly into the umbilical artery through the baby's umbilical cord.

Umbilical venous catheter (UVC)
A line placed directly into the umbilical vein (a much larger vein than a peripheral vein) through the baby's umbilical cord.

Varicella (chickenpox)
Common childhood illness characterized by an itchy rash and fever. When contracted by a pregnant woman, it can occasionally cause birth defects or severe illness in the baby. Varicella is highly contagious.

Vein
A blood vessel leading toward the heart.

Ventilator
Mechanical breathing machine.

Ventricle
A small chamber, one of the central chambers in the brain, or one of the 2 lower chambers of the heart.

Very low birth weight
Babies who are born weighing less than 1,500 g (3 lb 5 oz).

Very preterm
Babies born between 28 and 32 weeks' gestation.

Viable
A baby is potentially able to survive.

Vital signs
Temperature, heart rate, respiratory rate, and blood pressure.

Women, Infants, and Children (WIC)
A nutrition program that helps pregnant women, new mothers, and young children eat well and stay healthy. It provides food or formula to parents of babies.

Resources for Families

Web Sites

American Academy of Pediatrics (www.aap.org)

- **HealthyChildren.org** (www.HealthyChildren.org)
- **Healthy Child Care America (HCCA)** (www.healthychildcare.org)
- **HCCA Safe Sleep Campaign** (www.healthychildcare.org/sids.html)
- **Section on Neonatal-Perinatal Medicine** (www.aap.org/perinatal)

Bright Futures (http://brightfutures.aap.org)

CaringBridge (www.caringbridge.org)

Cystic Fibrosis Foundation (www.cff.org/AboutCF)

March of Dimes (www.marchofdimes.org)

- **Common conditions treated in the NICU** (www.marchofdimes.org/complications/common-conditions-treated-in-the-nicu.aspx)
- **Pregnancy** (www.marchofdimes.org/pregnancy/pregnancy.aspx)
- **Share Your Story** (www.shareyourstory.org)

National Association of Neonatal Nurses (www.nann.org)

Vaccines & Immunizations (www.cdc.gov/vaccines)

Books

Understanding the NICU: What Parents of Preemies and Other Hospitalized Newborns Need to Know, by Jeanette Zaichkin, RN, MN, NNP-BC, Editor in Chief; Gary Weiner, MD, FAAP, Contributing Editor; and David Loren, MD, FAAP, Contributing Editor

Parenting Your Premature Baby and Child: The Emotional Journey, by Deborah L. Davis, PhD, and Mara Tesler Stein, PsyD

Preemies: The Essential Guide for Parents of Premature Babies, 2nd Edition, by Dana Wechsler Linden, Emma Trenti Paroli, and Mia Wechsler Doron, MD

The Preemie Parents' Companion: The Essential Guide to Caring for Your Premature Baby in the Hospital, at Home, and Through the First Years, by Susan L. Madden, MS